Health Care Reform and Globalisation

The US, China and Europe in Comparative Perspective

Edited by
Peggy Watson

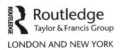
Routledge
Taylor & Francis Group

LONDON AND NEW YORK

First published 2013
by Routledge
2 Park Square, Milton Park, Abingdon, Oxon OX14 4RN

Simultaneously published in the USA and Canada
by Routledge
711 Third Avenue, New York, NY10017

Routledge is an imprint of the Taylor & Francis Group, an informa business

First issued in paperback 2014

British Library Cataloguing in Publication Data
A catalogue record for this book is available from the British Library

Library of Congress Cataloging in Publication Data
Health care reform and globalisation : the US, China, and Europe in comparative perspective / edited by Peggy Watson.
p. ; cm. -- (Routledge advances in health and social policy)
Includes bibliographical references.
I. Watson, Margaret, 1948- II. Series: Routledge advances in health and social policy.
[DNLM: 1. Health Care Reform--China. 2. Health Care Reform--Europe. 3. Health Care Reform--United States. 4. Internationality--China. 5. Internationality--Europe. 6. Internationality--United States. 7. Insurance, Health--China. 8. Insurance, Health--Europe. 9. Insurance, Health--United States. 10. National Health Programs--China. 11. National Health Programs--Europe. 12. National Health Programs--United States. WA 530 AA1]
362.1--dc23
2012003932

ISBN: 978-0-415-69108-6 (hbk)
ISBN: 978-0-203-10678-5 (ebk)

Typeset in Goudy
by Taylor & Francis Books

Health Care Reform and Globalisation

WITHDRAWN

In the post-Cold War, post-financial crisis era, health care is an issue of critical political, personal and economic concern. In the USA, plans to address a troubled health care model were met by vocal opposition. In the UK and post-communist Europe, attempts to introduce aspects of that model have resulted in controversy and violent protests, while China and Russia have recently introduced policies to counter the effects of marketising reforms. This innovative book provides a timely analysis addressing the many dimensions of radical health care change.

Bringing together three major geopolitical regions with strikingly different recent histories, this international cast of contributors examines reform in the USA, China and Europe within a single study frame. They look at the processes that have been involved when countries with such diverse starting points try to move towards a globally shared health care framework. An underlying theme running through the chapters is access to care, and how it is shaped by political and economic power, by moral economics, and by what can be said and known.

Health Care Reform and Globalisation confronts the interpretations and experiences of health care transformation in practice by patients, professionals and politicians. It will be of interest to scholars from a range of diverse disciplinary backgrounds, including public health, anthropology, area studies, sociology, politics, social policy, geography and economics.

Peggy Watson is at the Department of Sociology, University of Cambridge, and a Fellow of Homerton College, Cambridge, UK.

Contents

List of figures and tables   vii
List of contributors   viii
Introductory remarks and acknowledgements   x
PEGGY WATSON

1   Producing public opinion: how the insurance industry
    shaped US health care   1
    WENDELL POTTER

2   The break-up of the NHS: implications for information
    systems   25
    ALLYSON POLLOCK AND DAVID PRICE

3   Rethinking problems surrounding access to care:
    the moral economies shaping health care
    workforces in Russia and the USA   40
    MICHELE RIVKIN-FISH

4   Human oriented? Angels and monsters in China's
    health care reform   71
    MEI ZHAN

5   We are all in this together – European policies and
    health systems change   93
    MERI KOIVUSALO

6   Catastrophic citizenship and discourses of
    disguise: aspects of health care change in Poland   118
    PEGGY WATSON

7   The making of health care policy in contemporary
    Hungary   139
    TERRY COX AND SANDOR GALLAI

8 Community health services in urban China: a geographical
case study of access to care 164
YU WANG, TANGHONG JIA, JINGHUI ZHANG, YUNLI ZHANG, WEN LI
AND ROBERT HAINING

9 'Health care and change': popular protest and building
alternative visions of health systems at the end of empire 182
HOWARD WAITZKIN AND REBECA JASSO-AGUILAR

Index 209

Figures and tables

Figures

7.1 The balance of the Health Insurance Fund 148
8.1 Challenges facing China's CHS system 173
8.2 (a) Map of types of residential area in Jinan City; (b) overlay map
of 800-metre buffer zones of CHS institutions in Jinan City 177

Tables

6.1 Households not seeking required care for financial reasons
2008–09, by socioeconomic category 125
8.1 CHS 800-metre buffer zone coverage by type of residential area 178

List of contributors

Terry Cox is Professor of Central and East European Studies at the University of Glasgow, UK, and Editor of *Europe–Asia Studies*.

Sándor Gallai is Associate Professor in the Institute of Political Science at Corvinus University, and head of the Institute for Public Policy Research, Budapest, Hungary.

Robert Haining is Professor of Human Geography at the Department of Geography, University of Cambridge, UK.

Rebeca Jasso-Aguilar is a PhD candidate and a 2009–12 Andrew W. Mellon Doctoral Fellow in the Department of Sociology, University of New Mexico, USA.

Tanghong Jia is Professor of Hand Surgery and head of the Jinan Municipal Health Bureau, Jinan, China.

Meri Koivusalo is Senior Researcher at the National Institute for Health and Welfare, Helsinki, Finland.

Wen Li is in the Division of Community Health Services, at the Jinan Municipal Health Bureau, Jinan, China.

Allyson Pollock is Professor of Public Health Research and Policy, and Co-Director of the Global Health, Policy and Innovation Unit, Centre for Primary Care and Public Health, at Queen Mary, University of London, UK.

Wendell Potter is former Vice-President of corporate communications at CIGNA, and currently a Senior Analyst at the Center for Public Integrity and a Fellow at the Center for Media Democracy, USA.

David Price is Senior Research Fellow in the Global Health, Policy and Innovation Unit, Centre for Primary Care and Public Health, at Queen Mary, University of London, UK.

Michele Rivkin-Fish is Associate Professor of Medical Anthropology at the University of North Carolina, USA.

Howard Waitzkin is Distinguished Professor Emeritus, Clinical Professor of Medicine, and 2010–12 Presidential Teaching Fellow, University of New Mexico, USA.

Yu Wang is a PhD candidate in the Department of Geography, University of Cambridge, UK.

Peggy Watson is at the Department of Sociology, University of Cambridge, and Fellow of Homerton College, Cambridge, UK.

Mei Zhan is Associate Professor of Anthropology at the University of California, Irvine, USA.

Jinghui Zhang is Director of the Division of Community Health Services at the Jinan Municipal Health Bureau, Jinan, China.

Yunli Zhang is Deputy Director of the Division of Community Health Services, at the Jinan Municipal Health Bureau, Jinan, China.

Introductory remarks and acknowledgements

This book brings together papers that were discussed at a meeting held at the Centre for Research in the Arts, Social Sciences and Humanities (CRASSH) at the University of Cambridge on 24–25 June 2011. The meeting had the generous support of the British Academy, the Foundation for the Sociology of Health and Illness, and CRASSH, for which thanks are due. I am indebted to Anna Malinowska, former conference coordinator at CRASSH, for originally encouraging the project, as well as to Helga Brandt and Ruth Rushworth of CRASSH for their incomparable skills in organising the event and making it run so smoothly. Many thanks of course go to all of the participants of the meeting for a vital and diverse set of papers, and for two days of lively, engaged and non-stop conversation, which made this such an interesting and memorable event.

I am grateful to Wendell Potter for bringing his insight and experience as a former communications executive in the US health insurance corporation CIGNA, as well as his knowledge of journalism, to give a unique insider's perspective on how corporations have influenced health care debate and policy in the United States. I thank Allyson Pollock for providing an understanding of the way academic standards are at risk in the struggle over what is to count as knowledge, and the way that knowledge is used to underpin official rhetoric of health care change in England – a struggle that was unfolding in the national press as the conference was taking place.

The conference project was prompted by the asymmetry characterising the way the radical health care changes taking place simultaneously in many parts of the world were reaching the public eye. Its purpose was to critically address the contradictions and connections in contemporary health care change by bringing the USA, China and Europe together within a single analytical frame.

In 2009 the western media were full of stories recounting the debate and vociferous conflict that surrounded Barack Obama's proposals for health care reform in the United States. Yet the profound health care changes that had been taking place elsewhere, particularly in post-socialist Europe, were being passed over in virtual silence – not only in the media, but in academic work.

Discussion of the proposals for reform in the United States had highlighted the extent of the social and economic problems caused by a largely private benefits system that had come apart in the previous two decades, leaving millions without coverage. The US health care system had become by far the most expensive in the world. Yet during those two decades, the ideology and many of the practices underpinning the troubled US health care system had been exported to the post-socialist world, largely on the grounds that such marketisation would increase efficiency and reduce costs.

What ensued in practice was escalating health care costs and hugely increasing inequalities of access in countries that – in contrast to the west – remained relatively poor. Spiralling costs were the corollary of the rising and often tax-free profits accruing to transnational corporations from the creation and exploitation of post-socialist health care markets. The changes proved unpopular with many people in the countries concerned. In the relative absence of genuine debate, resistance took diverse forms, including opinion poll outcomes, health-worker strikes and street protests. The 2012 protests across Romania, which were sparked by health care privatisation proposals, were said to be the most violent the country had witnessed since 1989.

China's route to health care liberalisation began in 1978, with a ten-year plan that focused resources on economic development. At this time, the country began to dismantle its previous health care system, putting nothing in its place. Concurrently, the US gained reinvigorated international ascendancy, as marketising globalisation gathered pace in the wake of the 1970s capitalist crisis in the west. China cut health care expenditure so severely that by 2000 it had among the lowest share of government spending on health seen anywhere in the world. Access to health care became massively unequal as, in the absence of funding, state hospitals began charging patients for treatment and drugs. After rural cooperatives were disbanded, many former barefoot doctors resorted to selling medicines at high cost. In the meantime, the number of private hospitals was increasing and small-scale private practice spread. This policy context was transformed by the advent of severe acute respiratory syndrome (SARS) in 2003. The prospect of a public health catastrophe brought home the extent to which liberalised health care had undermined public health information systems and infrastructure, and had weakened the government's ability to act. Six years later, in 2009, the government announced a very substantial increase in the provision of health care and the intention to make basic health care universal by 2020.

The chapters in this volume are written from diverse disciplinary perspectives, including anthropology, sociology, geography, area studies and public health. The aim was to reflect – and connect – the many registers in which health care change can be understood. A recurrent theme in individual book chapters relates to how what can be said and known shapes, and is shaped by, ideologies, practices and debates. Wendell Potter, for example, discusses how much of the public furore surrounding Obama's proposed health care reforms was fuelled by stealth PR tactics funded to the tune of millions by corporations. Stealth campaigns engaged a politics of fear by encouraging people to see increased health coverage as a threat. Potter also discusses the extent to which government was disabled in debate by lack of access to the actuarial data which, under the US system, was held uniquely in private hands. Conversely, Allyson Pollock and David Price highlight the loss of public health information that will be the consequence of the introduction of elements of the US-style health maintenance organisation system planned for England. Public health information, previously collated on the basis of geographically defined populations, will be lost as it is replaced by the insurance pool-based data held by private firms. Meanwhile, China's efforts to put in place a geographically based system of community health centres, among others, because of what was learned concerning the immediate threat posed by lack of public health data and infrastructure during the trauma of SARS, is described on the basis of a case study of Jinan city by Yu Wang and his colleagues. The Chinese reforms also sought to address the mistrust that has been created as a result of the dismantling of health care. As Mei Zhan shows in her chapter, that mistrust had come to focus explicitly on doctors who, in the eyes of the public, had become the personification of greed.

Michele Rivkin-Fish brings to the surface the fundamental, but often submerged, forms of knowledge that sustain unequal access to health care. She does this by introducing the concept of moral economies to the study of health care policy in Russia and the United States. Moral economies involve unspoken understandings of entitlement that influence judgements about which claims are legitimate – leaving other needs unrecognised. Drawing on her ethnographic work in both countries, Rivkin-Fish highlights the complexity of what is involved in the pursuit of more equal health care access. Examining the moral economies of health care and professional work through which providers in Russia and the United States make sense of their career decisions and daily practice, she suggests, will open up new ways of seeing the challenges involved in widening access to include underserved populations. Peggy Watson discusses the events and processes through which health care changes that centre on privatisation have been pursued in Poland, highlighting the processes through which marketisers have drawn on symbolic distinctions between modernity and backwardness to discursively legitimate the effects of markets, and to promote markets in health care through the creation of a political economy of shame.

The book closes with a chapter by Howard Waitzkin and Rebeca Jasso-Aguilar, in which they suggest that Latin America is a prime site of resistance to the neoliberal health care pursued globally by the USA by virtue of the knowledge gained from their particular experience of exploitation. The authors suggest that we are reaching the end of empire – that is, the era of US world dominance is drawing to a close. The chapters in this book focus on health care changes that have occurred during the period of US-dominated neoliberal globalisation set in train in the 1970s, and especially the period of intensified globalisation that took place after the Cold War came to an end.

The extent to which that trajectory of social change continues depends not just on critical engagement with its effects, but also on the consequences for global power relations of the current crisis of capitalism.

Peggy Watson
Department of Sociology
University of Cambridge

1 Producing public opinion: how the insurance industry shaped US health care

Wendell Potter

The American health system is the most expensive in the world.[1] It is also one of the most inequitable. Hospitals in major metropolitan areas are gleaming cathedrals of technology. But by some very meaningful measures, the American health system itself is sick, lagging behind far less developed countries. According to a frequently cited World Health Organization study, a baby born in Bosnia has a longer life expectancy than one born in the United States of America. The citizens of Bangladesh have more equitable access to health care than their American counterparts. The United States ranks 47th in life expectancy at birth and 54th in fairness, a measure of the extent to which the best care is available equally throughout a country (WHO 2000). Nearly 51 million Americans have no health care coverage, and, according to the Commonwealth Fund, an additional 25 million are considered underinsured. Many in low-paying jobs have only the illusion of health care coverage (DeNavas-Walt et al. 2010). The number of uninsured and underinsured Americans has grown larger as for-profit corporations have come to dominate the health insurance industry. At the same time, the percentage of premiums that insurers spend paying claims, reflected by an equation called the medical loss ratio (MLR), has steadily declined. The higher the MLR, the more the insurer has paid out in claims. From 1993 to 2010, the average MLR, which is a key measure that investors consider in evaluating an insurer's financial performance, dropped from 95 percent to around 80 percent. Investors prefer to see a decreasing MLR every quarter, and if they don't, their displeasure can be reflected in a decrease in the company's stock price.

It was in this environment, in 2008, that Barack Obama was elected President of the United States. His election was thanks, in part, to his stance on health care reform. Indeed, many health care reform advocates in the United States believed the stars had aligned for a fundamental restructuring of the American health care system with Obama's election and the Democrats' firm control of both chambers of Congress. Health care had been a major campaign issue, and many advocates believed Obama would succeed in shepherding legislation through Congress that would bring about radical changes in how care is financed and delivered in the United States, and that would guarantee universal coverage. As it turned out, they underestimated the ability of entrenched special interests, especially health insurers, to influence the legislative process by skillful manipulation of public opinion.

The basics of health care in the United States

In the United States, health care coverage comes in a variety of forms. Americans use private coverage both as a way to insulate themselves from the prohibitive costs of medical care for a catastrophic illness, and to grant them access to other necessary health care services. A wide array of public and private sources provide health coverage. Public sources include Medicare, Medicaid, the State Children's Health Insurance Program, federal and state employee health plans, the military and the Veterans Administration.[2] In very basic terms, most Americans with health care coverage get it through their employer. This coverage comes through either a state-licensed health insuring organization or a self-funded employee health benefit plan that operates under federal law and is sponsored by an employer or an employee organization.

Citizens aged 65 and older, and younger citizens with permanent disabilities, are most commonly enrolled in Medicare as their health insurance program. Established in 1965, it consists of four parts: Part A covers hospital expenses; Part B pays for doctor visits, outpatient care, and home health; Part C, the Medicare Advantage program, allows beneficiaries to enroll in a private plan; and Part D covers prescription drugs. Medicare does not, however, cover many relatively expensive services and supplies, long-term care (whether in the patient's home or at an assisted living facility), or nursing homes. How these coverage options were arrived at, and what their fate will be in the years to come, tells a great deal of the story of reform efforts in the United States, and how those efforts have been affected by the furtive application of influence over the public by powerful special interests and the often shadowy organizations they deploy.

How special interests used propaganda and often stealth public relations campaigns to shape the development of the US health care system

Public relations has become a great force in the United States in shaping public opinion and, ultimately, public policy. The use of often secretive PR tactics began in earnest soon after the turn of the twentieth century, when business leaders such as John D. Rockefeller, who were frequently the subject of critical news coverage, hired former newspaper reporters to help them enhance their reputations. Tobacco companies were also among the first clients of the early PR practitioners in the USA. One of the big tobacco companies even hired a PR firm in the 1920s, in a successful effort to persuade young women that smoking was not just for men, that it was in fact a fashionable and liberating thing to do. When the tobacco industry found itself in a fight for survival in the 1960s, after the US Surgeon General declared that smoking caused cancer and other often fatal illnesses, it hired big PR firms to cast doubt on the government's findings. And when cigarette makers came under fire for encouraging smoking among minors, and studies emerged about second-hand smoke, they hired their own scientists to spin messages about the beneficial effects of tobacco.

The industry also recruited a wide range of 'soft scientists' – sociologists, philosophers, political scientists, psychologists, and economists – to influence public opinion through cultural routes. For example, the industry recruited economists to produce 'studies' based on non-scientific, anecdotal evidence that claimed to demonstrate how bans on smoking hurt businesses. The science was weak, but the dissemination process was comprehensive. For decades, whenever there was a public push for a law restricting smoking in restaurants, restaurant owners would claim they were afraid of losing business, citing those commissioned reports. One prominent philosopher, while secretly taking payments from Japan Tobacco, wrote articles deriding public health advocacy and publishing pro-smoking stories in newspapers and international magazines (Kmietowicz and Ferriman 2002). He coined the term 'nanny state' – a phrase still regularly employed by politicians – claimed that seat belt laws caused people to drive faster, extolled the benefits of risk-taking, and argued that smoking was actually a healthy activity because of its stress-relieving benefits.

What the tobacco industry essentially was doing during this time was creating a primer on how corporations and their trade associations could use stealth PR to manipulate public opinion and influence public policy without anyone being aware of the true sponsors of the PR initiatives. Indeed, the tobacco industry's PR strategies have been so broadly based, well funded, effective, and replicable that they comprise a kind of PR 'playbook' to which almost all industries, including the health insurance industry, turn when under attack.

Reform attempts from the 1940s to the 1970s – and how PR campaigns ended most of them

In 1945, President Franklin Roosevelt died, the Second World War ended, and Harry S. Truman became the first president in the nation's history openly to endorse a single universal comprehensive health insurance plan. Truman's first major peacetime address to Congress, in November 1945, laid out his agenda. In announcing his legislative proposal Truman noted that during the Second World War, nearly 5 million Americans had been classified as unfit for military service for health reasons, and another 3 million had been trea-ted or discharged for physical or mental problems that had existed before their induction. 'In the past,' he told Congress, 'the benefits of modern medical science have not been enjoyed by our citizens with any degree of equality. Nor are they today. Nor will they be in the future unless government is bold enough to do something about it. We should resolve now that the health of this nation is a national concern; that financial barriers in the way of attaining health shall be removed; that the health of all its citizens deserves the help of all the nation' (Daschle 2008: 49).

The American Medical Association (AMA) – which had opposed medical reform in previous decades as 'an incitement to revolution' – cast Truman's 'socialized medicine' as an extension of Russian communistic control of the world. The AMA's *Journal* wrote: '(If this) Old World scourge is allowed to spread to our New World, (it will) jeopardize the health of our people and gravely endanger our freedom' (Henderson 1949). Republicans in the House blocked the bill from even getting a hearing. The press took up the AMA's argument that the legislation would make doctors 'slaves.' Truman responded that it allowed doctors to choose their own form of payment. Not only did the legislation not advance in 1946, the Republicans used it against the Democrats and Truman's 'socialism,' and swept back into control of Congress in that fall's elections.

The pendulum quickly swung back the other way when Truman made public health care part of his own re-election platform in 1948, and staged one of the biggest election upsets in US history, also leading the Democrats back into power on Capitol Hill. The AMA asked of each of its members an additional $25 and hired a PR firm (Whitaker & Baxter) as part of an anti-Truman campaign in 1949. The campaign against Truman cost $1.5 million, more than had ever been spent before on such an effort (Starr 1982: 285). Part of the PR effort was a poster and a pamphlet distributed to patients in doctors' waiting rooms across the country that proclaimed, 'The Voluntary Way is the American Way.' The AMA also enlisted as allies insurers and employers as part of a *quid pro quo* in which the AMA urged its own members to ask patients to purchase private, voluntary insurance to head off the attempt to enslave them. The US Chamber of Commerce printed a pamphlet of its own, called *You and Socialized Medicine*, that urged member companies to endorse and purchase private group-insurance plans for their workers to eliminate any need for a public plan. Southern politicians also joined the opposition by preaching at home that the dangers of 'socialized' medicine included an end to racially segregated hospitals and the enforcement of staff privileges for black doctors. This was the first-ever all-out paranoid-propaganda blitz by the country's health care sector (Daschle 2008: 53).

But it was the Soviet Union's establishment of a Communist government in East Germany, and the ascendancy of Mao Tse-tung's Communist party in the People's Republic of China, that finally dealt Truman's plan its death blow. As the Cold War began, Democrats retained control of Congress in the 1950 elections, but the GOP (the Republican 'Grand Old Party') made enough gains to stop any further effort by Truman to get national health insurance back on the agenda. Truman wrote later in his memoirs:

I cautioned Congress against being frightened away from health insurance by the scare words 'socialized medicine,' which some people were bandying about. I wanted no part of socialized medicine, and I knew the American people did not. I have had some stormy times as President and have engaged in some vigorous controversies. Democracy thrives on debate and political differences. But I had no patience with the reactionary selfish people and politicians who fought year after year every proposal we made to improve the people's health (Daschle 2008: 53).

The AMA's opposition to Truman, and its successful partnership with business and private-pay insurance companies, put into motion the market forces that eventually took control of American health care. As General Motors and other large employers began paying for health insurance and pensions for their workers in 1950, a shift was under way.

The 1950s were a prosperous decade for large for-profit insurance providers in the USA. It was during these years that commercial insurers began cherry-picking young and healthy premium-payers by offering them lower prices. Large employers began to self-insure by entering into tailored agreements with insurance carriers, thus no longer needing to belong to the health plans administered primarily by the non-profit Blue Cross and Blue Shield companies. By the end of the decade, insurers were 'experience rating' firms to base premiums on their employees' usage of services. All of these forces produced a golden age for the idea of free-market insurance. By 1963, nearly 80 percent of Americans were employer insured, and health care costs had largely been contained by market conditions.

Johnson and the creation of Medicare

By the 1960s, however, the nation's elderly were an increasing problem for the free-market paradigm because of their health care demands. Company health plans with benefits to retirees – mostly through unions – had to raise current workers' premiums in order to cover rising costs. The elderly without retiree benefits, including many who were poor and uninsured, were creating larger demands on state and local charity suppliers. The American health care solution was showing its Achilles heel. When the first legislation to cover hospital costs for people on Social Security was introduced in 1958, the AMA carried out the same paranoid-style attacks as before, but this time the tactic did not work as well. By concentrating their focus on problems of the aged, proponents of reform eventually passed a bill in 1960. The Kerr–Mills Act made federal grants available to the states to help them pay for health care for the elderly poor. However, only twenty-eight states signed onto the plan, and many of them didn't set aside enough state money to trigger the release of the federal funds. Many doctors and hospitals rejected payments because they were 'below the prevailing rate' (Daschle 2008: 59).

For the first time in US history, there was a groundswell of authentic grass-roots support for a tougher law. By 1962, polls were showing that 69 percent of Americans favored such a measure – by now called Medicare – and

President John F. Kennedy joined in the support, making it a legislative priority. The AMA created a political action committee, AMPAC, which recruited the personal doctors of members of Congress to lobby against the effort. It also ran newspaper, radio, and TV ads decrying Medicare as socialized medicine. The legislation lost by narrow votes in the first round, which gave Kennedy encouragement to introduce it again the following year. Although it had stalled the Medicare bill, the AMA for the first time began losing some of its partners, notably the American Hospital Association and some of the now-powerful for-profit insurance companies, who saw the effect of elderly health costs on their own bottom lines. With support from labor unions, too, and nearly universal support from elderly Americans, the Medicare idea was gaining steam when, in November 1963, Kennedy was assassinated and Lyndon Johnson assumed the presidency. Aided by the shock of Kennedy's death and the landslide victory of Johnson and the Democrats in 1964, Medicare was shoved across the finish line in 1965, though not before some final tweaks and compromises.

Realizing its losing position, the AMA lobbied for what it called Eldercare, an amplified version of the Kerr–Mills Act. Insurance companies, led by Aetna, pushed for another version, called Bettercare, which would provide federal money to be used for private health insurance premiums for the poor and elderly. In the final showdown, Wilbur Mills, House Ways and Means Committee chairman, combined all three ideas into the final Medicare bill, which he called his 'three-layer cake': Part A, which covered hospitals; Part B, which covered doctors and was optional; and Medicaid, a separate program for the states. Prescription drugs were not covered, nor were eyeglasses, dentists, or long-term care, but the final bill emerged as the largest expansion of health care coverage in American history. In a special homage to Truman, Johnson signed the bill on July 30, 1965, in Independence, Missouri, with Truman at his side.

> 'No longer will older Americans be denied the healing miracle of modern medicine,' Johnson said in signing the bill. 'No longer will illness crush and destroy the savings that they have so carefully put away over a lifetime so that they might enjoy dignity in their later years. No longer will young families see their own incomes, and their own hopes, eaten away simply because they are carrying out their deep moral obligations to their parents, and to their uncles, and their aunts ...'
>
> (quoted in Daschle 2008: 63).

Senator Kennedy's missed opportunity

The implementation of Medicare and Medicaid consumed enormous attention in government and the health care world for the next several years, but by 1970, growing health care costs and increased numbers of uninsured Americans among the non-elderly renewed the debate about more far-reaching health care reform. President Richard Nixon sounded the alarm, saying, 'We face a massive crisis in this area. Unless action is taken within the next two or three years … we will have a breakdown in our medical system.' The normally conservative media, including *Business Week* and *Fortune* magazines, supported him. Both had cover stories and special issues declaring that American medicine stood 'on the brink of chaos.' Polls also showed that 75 percent of American households agreed there was a 'crisis' (Starr 1982: 381).

Not satisfied with Nixon's approach to reform, Senator Ted Kennedy, chairman of the Senate Health Subcommittee, renewed the idea of national health insurance in 1971. Nixon responded with a private sector-based plan that would mandate employer health coverage for all working Americans, and would require employers offering traditional indemnity coverage to also offer a prepaid group plan called, for the first time, a health maintenance organization (HMO). Twenty-two different bills were circulating in Congress in 1971, ranging from Kennedy's comprehensive single-payer plan to a complicated but conservative scheme called Medicredit, supported by the AMA (Quadagno 2005: 116). Because of the number of proposals and the ephemeral nature of political alliances, Congress took no action on any bill in 1971 or 1972, an election year. The only plan to find common ground and get passed in 1973 was Nixon's Health Maintenance Organization and Resources Development Act (HMO Act), which required companies with twenty-five or more employees to provide an HMO option.

Kennedy and Mills eventually joined in a compromise bill that had the best potential. But soon thereafter, Mills was brought down by a sex scandal and Nixon resigned after Watergate. As a consequence, the compromise bill languished. Before he resigned, however, in the swirl of all the plans circulating, Nixon had actually offered a universal health care plan. Democrats opposed it, however. They wanted to hold out for a bill more to their liking, which they believed would eventually emerge and have broad public support. But nothing better ever came. In an article in *The Washington Post* in 2003, Senator Kennedy said that he regretted his decision thirty years earlier not to consider Nixon's plan. 'In retrospect,' he said, 'I'd grab that' (Dionne 2003).

The Clinton plan – and how deceptive PR efforts doomed it

When Bill Clinton became President of the United States in 1992, he promised to overhaul the health care system without expanding government or raising taxes. Momentum seemed to be with him. Mainstream media and political figures spoke of the Health Security initiative as if it were a *fait accompli*. Polls showed widespread public anxiety about access to adequate health care, and health costs were rising at the then unheard-of annual rate of 8.5 percent.[3] Conditions appeared favorable. By the time Clinton assumed office, however, a special-interest coalition comprising the chief executives of fifty insurance carriers, hospitals, drug companies, and medical-device manufacturers had been created. The CEOs had formed their group, which they called the Healthcare Leadership Council (HLC), initially to lobby the George H. W. Bush White House for reform favorable to them. Bush, who lost to Clinton in the 2000 presidential election, was not interested in their reform ideas, but the HLC stayed in business. For the first few months of the Clinton administration, there was a kind of uneasy honeymoon with the HLC, because of Clinton's indication that his legislation would be based on 'managed competition,' which, to the private-sector creators of the concept, meant minimal government involvement.

But within weeks of his inauguration, it became clear that the President and First Lady Hilary Clinton were considering more regulation of the insurance industry, as well as federally imposed spending caps to control rising health care costs. Insurance executives and their allies wasted no time attacking price controls, calling them a 'top-down' approach that would amount to 'rationing by chaos … a trap to be avoided at all costs' (PR Newswire 1992).

By the time the Clintons unveiled their plan several months later, the insurers were already on the attack, visibly and behind the scenes. Insurance executives lamented that the Clintons' reform legislation 'shed many essential free-market principles upon which managed competition functions.' The White House plan was hindered by its intimidating scope and complexity. It was seen as overly academic and an expansion of governmental authority, and concocted behind closed doors. As it was without precedent, the administration had difficulty comparing it with anything that people recognized. It involved state-level mandatory purchasing cooperatives, global budgets to limit total spending on health care, and caps on health insurance premiums. The Clintons also wanted to create a federal council to review prices for new drugs, and they wanted drug companies to pay rebates to the Medicare program.

The HLC, acting as a coalition for the special interests it represented, launched a multi-pronged attack that included grassroots organizing, lobbying by corporate executives, and PR efforts. It ran ads around the country raising the specter of health care rationing and warning of bureaucratic interference with patients' rights (Stone 1994). All of this was done under the name of the HLC, not the individual companies that funded it. The HLC described itself as 'the exclusive forum for the nation's health care leaders to jointly develop policies, plans, and programs to achieve their vision of a 21st century system that makes affordable, high-quality care accessible to all Americans.' In reality, what the HLC was lobbying for was fewer government regulations. One of its initial goals was to exempt employers of all sizes from state insurance mandates. Industry trade associations supplemented the HLC's efforts. TV ads sponsored by the Health Insurance Association of America featured a middle-aged, middle-class couple sitting at their kitchen table worrying about the new regulations. Radio ads warned that the Clintons' plan could lead to 'Washington bureaucrats deciding how much care can be given to you and your family.' The ads encouraged listeners to call a toll-free number to tell Congress that they opposed the Clinton plan. When callers dialed the number, they reached a 'grassroots' lobbying firm that patched the calls through to members of Congress. At the peak of the ad campaign, about 5000 calls a day were being generated, according to one of the leaders of the HLC.

By early fall of 1994, shortly after the HLC's radio campaign ended, the Clinton plan was officially dead. Senate majority leader George Mitchell pulled the plug on reform when it became clear he would never have enough votes in the Senate to overcome a filibuster. 'The $300 million that the health insurance and other lobbies had spent to stop health care reform was well invested,' Clinton wrote ten years later in his memoir (Clinton 2004: 62). Without energetic support in Congress, the initiative simply ran out of political and parliamentary steam. 'The president and his allies could have done a better job than they did of explaining the regulatory mechanisms in their plan,' wrote Harvard University sociologist Theda Skocpol in *Health Affairs*.

> But even if the Clinton administration had communicated more effectively, the plan might still have gone down to a defeat that backfired badly against the Democrats. The bedrock fact is that the Clinton plan promised too much cost-cutting regulation and not enough payoffs to organized groups and middle-class citizens pleasantly ensconced in the existing U.S. health care system (Skocpol 1995).

And that November, the political bill for Clinton's miscalculations came due. Riding a wave of anti-government sentiment that the health care reform battle had aroused, Republicans took advantage of an anaemic Democratic turnout and won control of the House for the first time in forty years, and the Senate for the first time since 1986.

In 1992, enactment of Clinton's plan had seemed to be inevitable. Just two years later, the health insurance industry walked unscathed out of the rubble of the collapse of that certainty. Instead of facing new regulations that threatened their business models, insurers faced conditions that were ideal for letting the 'invisible hand' of capitalism spread their aggressive management of medical care across the country – and create enormous profits in the process. Nowhere was this clearer than when the Blue Cross and Blue Shield Association, a trade group for non-profit health insurers, amended its bylaws to permit members to convert into public-stock companies (Wynn 1996). The change refocused health plans away from local service and non-profit status. They were now able to consolidate into for-profit, national entities that would eventually drive many smaller local competitors out of business or force them to sell out to larger companies. Fourteen Blue Cross plans, most of which dominated their statewide markets, converted from non-profits into for-profits, and by 2004 they had all become wholly owned subsidiaries of WellPoint, a large holding company. About one-third of nearly 100 million Blue Cross subscribers in the United States now belong to a for-profit plan operated by WellPoint, which has the biggest enrollment of any private insurer.

The Obama plan

On March 23, 2010, after more than a year of contentious debate and often raucous town hall meetings across the country, President Obama signed the Patient Protection and Affordable Care Act. At more than 2000 pages long, it represented the most sweeping changes in the American health care system since Lyndon Johnson's Medicare program. The bill that reached his desk, however, was not the one that many reform advocates had been hoping for. They believed that the President and Congressional leaders had capitulated to the insurance industry and its allies on too many important issues. The road to getting any law passed had been a punishing one, a road on which not one inch of progress was made without political turmoil. The public debate was a noisy one, and actual discussion of issues was often difficult to hear. Two catchphrases in particular – 'government takeover' and 'death panels' – not only did much to derail it, but in the months leading up to Obama's signing, they shaped the debate about the proposed health care law.

Frank Luntz, a Republican strategist, encouraged use of the term 'government takeover,' with its images of government bureaucrats determining health care in grey, state-run institutions. In a twenty-eight-page memo entitled 'The Language of Healthcare 2009,' Luntz wrote, 'Takeovers are like coups. They both lead to dictators and a loss of freedom.'[4] Echoing characterizations of Medicare in the 1960s and the Clinton plan in the 1990s, the line was picked up by lawmakers and pundits, and may have done more to ensure the government-run public option Obama had championed during his campaign was left out of the legislation. The phrase appeared more than ninety times on House Speaker John Boehner's website, GOPLeader.gov; eight times in 'A Pledge to America,' the Republican 2010 campaign platform; and more than 200 times on the Republican National Committee's website.[5] Within the public debate, it achieved the status of fact. Luntz's memo stressed that, when arguing against the bill, the discussion 'must center around politicians, bureaucrats and Washington.' The memo was followed, the messages were repeated, and by the time Obama signed the bill into law, 53 percent of respondents in a Bloomberg poll agreed that the bill 'amounts to a government takeover.'[6] The 'death panel' phrase was born on Sarah Palin's Facebook page. Palin's coining of the term was inspired by former New York Lieutenant Governor Betsy McCaughey, who, on July 16, 2009, claimed in a commentary that there was a provision in the proposed legislation in which 'Congress would make it mandatory ... that, every five years, people in Medicare have a required counseling session that will tell them how to end their life sooner, how to decline nutrition' (Begley 2009). The provision McCaughey was mis-characterizing was in a House bill. It would have required that Medicare cover optional counseling, upon request by the patient, about end-of-life care. 'Death panels,' as a phrase and as a political tool, was clear, easy to remember, and effective. Again, while proponents of health care reform talked about tens of millions of uninsured Americans, and used often lengthy explanations of the plan and why it was needed, health care reform opponents rarely varied from their succinct talking points, which were designed to create fear of reform.

The rhetoric was a testament to the power of a good investment. Health insurers and other groups invested in front groups that not only spawned such phrases as 'government takeover,' but continually turned the debate to questions of patriotism, and went so far as to employ racist images and slogans. Lobbyists, whose ranks also included former House majority leader Dick Armey of Texas, mounted protests that led to the formation of the Tea Party (Good 2009). As the struggle began for control of the provisions that would find their way into the bill, opponents of reform had many goals, but one imperative: to kill a proposed government-administered 'public option.'

Beating back the public option

When Obama officially kicked off the health care reform debate in a March 2009 summit, just weeks after being sworn into office, one of the people among the 150 invited guests was the health insurance industry's point person in Washington, Karen Ignagni, president of America's Health Insurance Plans (AHIP), the largest trade group of private health insurers. The softly spoken Ignagni was the public face of an $800 billion-a-year industry, and her mission was to ensure to the extent possible that reform would benefit insurers and result in minimal additional regulations on the industry. At the March summit, she promised the President that insurers would work with him and Congress to pass health care reform. Behind the scenes, however, AHIP already had begun to unleash a sophisticated, multi-pronged attack to undermine it.

From 2007 to mid-2009, insurance and HMO political contributions and lobbying expenses totaled $586 million, according to the Center for Responsive Politics, a non-partisan group dedicated to overhauling US campaign finance laws.[7] At the height of the political battle, the industries that would be most directly affected by reform were spending nearly $700,000 a day to influence the process.[8]

Meanwhile, in the House of Representatives, leaders reached consensus on the creation of a public option to function as a formidable competitor to private companies in the reformed health insurance marketplace. The public option was the brainchild of Yale political science professor Jacob Hacker, whose arguments were detailed and compelling (Hacker 2008). Progressive activists, consumer advocates, labor unions – and their newly formed umbrella group, Health Care for America Now (HCAN) – embraced the public option as the only way to force millions of new customers to buy health insurance without creating a public backlash.

Liberals generally held that a national public option would be the best way to curb soaring health care costs. The most prominent public plan, Medicare, had recorded annual spending growth lower than private insurers' over the previous decade with per capita costs growing by 4.4 percent a year under Medicare versus 7.4 percent under private health insurance.[9] It was precisely this superior cost-control performance that made so many health care providers, from pharmaceutical companies to doctors and hospitals, leery of health care reform. They worried that a public option would underpay them and take away their power to charge 'what the traffic would bear'. Eventually, in return for their not attacking reform, the drug and hospital industries negotiated deals with the Obama administration that locked in limits on their own health care reform concessions.

Insurers worried, with good reason, that they would not be able to compete against a government-run plan that could offer lower premiums because it would not need to make a profit or spend as much as private plans on marketing and sales activities. In April 2009, when it became clear that the House bill likely would include a public option, The Lewin Group (a forty-year-old health-policy consulting firm that had been acquired two years earlier by UnitedHealth, one of the largest health insurers in the USA) released a report suggesting that a public option would force 119 million Americans out of their employer-sponsored health plans and into the government insurance plan.[10] Republicans eagerly embraced the claim, even though the Lewin report was not based on any actual legislation. A July 23, 2009 story in *The Washington Post* quoted a Lewin Vice-President acknowledging that Americans would not be forced into a government-run plan if a public option were created, and that many people 'might very well be better off' if they could choose between a government-run plan and private options (Hilzenrath 2009). After its analysis had been widely questioned, Lewin reduced its estimate of the impact of the public option to 'only' 88.1 million people. Soon thereafter, the non-partisan CBO found that the public option would draw only 11 million people from the 170 million covered by private health plans. But the 119 million figure had been circulating for weeks, and opponents continued to use Lewin's disputed public option projections as supporting evidence that Obama and congressional leaders were bent on a 'government takeover' of the health care system.

Using its vast information technology resources, the industry was in the advantageous position of providing actuarial data to those who were considering the bill. Virtually no-one on Capitol Hill had the background or skills to question the evidence. Congressional staffers at the highest levels of the discussions confessed that they had to ask insurance companies themselves for comparative actuarial analyses of various scenarios to help formulate proposals for members of Congress. Congressional offices had no access to the actual data, and could not run such research independently. *Business Week* captured the effectiveness of that approach in a cover story on August 6, 2009. 'UnitedHealth,' the magazine reported, 'has distinguished itself by more deftly and aggressively feeding sophisticated pricing and actuarial data to information-starved Congressional staff members. With its rivals, the carrier has also achieved a secondary aim of constraining the new benefits that will become available to tens of millions of people who are currently uninsured. That will make the new customers more lucrative to the industry' (Terhune and Epstein 2009).

The rough road to reform

Health Care for America Now (HCAN), the umbrella group for most reform advocates, would spend more than $47 million on health care reform, its money coming from member contributions and grants from private foundations, most notably The Atlantic Philanthropies. According to HCAN's leader, long-time organizer and activist Richard Kirsch, 'We represent the deepest single-issue coalition in modern American history.' HCAN's aim was to support centrist Democrats, especially freshmen and conservative incumbents from districts where Obama had fared poorly in the election. In addition to spending millions of dollars for TV ads, HCAN made use of an unprece-dented progressive activist base, with the help of coalition members such as the AFL-CIO (American Federation of Labor and Congress of Industrial Organizations), MoveOn.org, the Service Employees International Union, the American Federation of State, County and Municipal Workers, Americans United for Change, the Center for Community Change, the American Federation of Teachers, Campaign for America's Future, True Majority, the United Food and Commercial Workers, and the Communications Workers of America. HCAN brought delegations of field partners to Congressional district offices, flooding their Washington offices with handwritten letters, arranging for leaders of local grassroots groups to visit members' offices, generating media coverage of protests and rallies, visiting newspaper editorial boards, releasing research reports, and organizing large-scale rallies. HCAN adopted a coordinating role that had, in fact, never been used on the left as it had on the right.

In July 2009, House leaders pushed a bill through three committees that included the public option and a surtax on high-income earners. To win the support of the more conservative Democrats, the leadership agreed to include certain tax exemptions for businesses. No Republicans voted for it in any of the committees. In the Senate, as Finance Committee meetings dragged on, reform advocates kept pressing forward, with a new ally. The American Medical Association, a crucial interest group, endorsed the public option – a far cry from its historical positions that had helped defeat reform for more than a century. In August, the month of Congress's recess, Karen Ignagni bluntly warned members of Congress not to blast her industry. She told the Associated Press that if lawmakers used the recess to vilify insurers, 'members of Congress will come back to Washington without a strong sense that health care reform is doable. And that would be a lost opportunity. We think health care reform is going to be won or lost in August.' Obama had begun talking by then about insurance company abuses and record profits, and Pelosi went so far as to call insurers 'villains.' Ignagni responded by saying that 'when polls are slipping, people turn to tried-and-true tactics.'[11]

Members of Congress were frequently greeted in town hall meetings by angry but often misinformed protesters. At numerous events, protesters carried signs demanding that the government keep its hands 'off my Medicare.' The irony, of course, is that Medicare is a government-run program.

Allies of the insurance industry had begun sending e-mails to millions of people with misleading and often false claims about the contents of pending bills, including the one about death panels. Polls showed that millions of people, especially seniors, believed the rumors. It was all part of a coordinated strategy. Many journalists based reports on memos from 'astroturf' (fake grassroots) groups – including Dick Armey's Freedom Works and Americans for Prosperity – that advised members on how to put Members of Congress on the defensive by disrupting presentations, and charging that Democrats were supporting a 'socialist agenda.'

After the summer recess, Obama tried to restore support for reform. During a speech before a joint session of Congress, he criticized his opponents' 'scare tactics' and made his strongest case yet for comprehensive reform. When he said that illegal immigrants would not be given health care coverage under any bill being considered by Congress, Representative Joe Wilson from South Carolina stunned his colleagues and visitors in the House chamber when he yelled, 'You lie!'. Wilson was soon thereafter rebuked by the House, and polls showed that Obama had stopped the slide in public opinion favoring reform. The following week, however, the bill that was finally reported out of the Senate Finance Committee did not include a public option, much to the disappointment of reform advocates. Insurers were pleased that they had been able to strip the public option out of the bill, but were unhappy that the penalties to be assessed against Americans who did not buy health insurance were, in their opinion, too low to be effective.

AHIP hired the accounting firm PriceWaterhouseCoopers (PwC) to produce a report showing that health care reform as envisioned by Senate Democrats would hurt most Americans rather than help them. The report predicted that reform would drive premiums up and require most Americans to pay an excise tax on their policies. The report contradicted the Congressional Budget Office as well as other independent experts, who concluded that insurance companies would respond to an excise tax on expensive health care plans by slowing the growth of health care costs. The White House immediately attacked the AHIP-funded report. 'It is hard to take it seriously,' said White House spokeswoman Linda Douglass. 'The analysis completely ignores critical policies that will lower costs for those who have insurance, expand coverage, and provide affordable health insurance options to millions of Americans who are priced out of today's health insurance market or are locked out by unfair insurance company practices.'[12]

The White House said it was blindsided by the report, that Ignagni herself had, just days before, assured administration officials that AHIP had no plans to launch an immediate attack on the Senate Finance Committee bill. The controversy became so intense that PwC backed away from its own findings, pointing out that it had focused only on the parts of health care reform that AHIP opposed – as AHIP had directed – while ignoring everything else. The uproar over the AHIP/PwC report briefly revived reform advocates' hopes of a public option (Murray and Montgomery 2009). Those hopes were short-lived, however. Democrats were shocked when a Republican came from behind to win a special January 2010 election in Massachusetts to replace Senator Ted Kennedy, who had died in August. The loss of that seat meant that the Democrats no longer had a filibuster-proof majority in the Senate. Not only was the public option in danger, so was comprehensive reform of any kind.

As Obama and stunned Democrats tried to figure out how to proceed, Anthem Blue Cross, California's largest health insurer, began notifying 800,000 of its customers that it was going to raise their premiums by as much as 39 percent (Helfand 2010). The move sparked a backlash that attracted national media attention. Obama, Health and Human Services Secretary Kathleen Sebelius, and Congressional Democrats seized on the planned rate increase and kept the story alive for days, overshadowing the Republicans' continuing efforts to kill what reform opponents were by now calling 'Obamacare'. There was also opposition within the Democratic Party, not the least of which was opposition to the legislation from a group of socially conservative Democrats who wanted to strengthen restrictions on abortions. At the other end of the philosophical spectrum, many liberals continued to insist on a public option. Reform advocates who had hoped reform would lead to a Canadian-style single payer system in the USA were so dismayed that many of them suggested that the Democrats should scuttle the Senate bill and start over. Obama warned the groups that continued delay would endanger not only reform, but also the Democrats' hopes of holding on to their majorities in Congress. After many closed-door meetings among Democratic leaders on Capitol Hill and at the White House, the Senate bill was passed, and Obama signed it into law.

Although the Patient Protection and Affordable Care Act (its official name) does achieve many of the reform advocates' goals – it will, among other things, expand the Medicaid program for low-income Americans to cover many more families; it will make it illegal for insurance companies to deny coverage because of pre-existing conditions; it will provide tax credits to small businesses to encourage them to offer health benefits to their employees; and it will enhance the prescription drug benefit for Medicare enrollees – it also met the insurance industry's objectives. The bill was enacted with the individual mandate, which Obama had opposed during his campaign, but without the public option, which he had endorsed and said early in the debate was an essential part of reform. While the law does impose numerous new regulations on the industry, they are not onerous for most insurers. In fact, 2010 was very profitable for the big publicly traded insurers, and, if their earnings for the first three months of this year are an indication, 2011 will be one of their most profitable years ever. So, in many ways, the reform law is just as beneficial to the insurance industry as it is to individual Americans – maybe even more beneficial.

Into the breach

A fact sheet published by the Obama administration last summer promised that '(t)he Affordable Care Act will help support and protect consumers and end some of the worst insurance company abuses.' It went on to assure us that the new rules would guarantee consumer access to both internal and external appeals processes 'that are clearly defined, impartial, and designed to ensure that, when health care is needed and covered, consumers get it.' – 'In implementing this law, we have worked to end the worst insurance company abuses, preserve existing options and slow premium increases,' an administration official said. 'Through it all, protecting consumers has been – and remains – our top priority.'[13]

Congress gave the National Association of (State) Insurance Commissioners (NAIC) the responsibility of writing many of the new regulations required by the new law. One of the regulations pertains to a section of the law that expands the rights of patients to appeal a coverage denial by an insurer. If the regulations are implemented as the NAIC recommends, many patients for the first time will be able to get an external appeal on a broad range of coverage denials, including denials that result from an insurer's decision to rescind, or cancel, a patient's policy – not just denials made on the basis of 'medical necessity' as determined by the insurer. The NAIC's standards also say that insurers must provide consumers with clear information about their rights to both internal and external appeals, and that the companies must expedite the appeals process in urgent or emergency situations.

Insurers are pushing back. Consumer advocates who have been in meetings at the White House to discuss the implementation of various provisions of the law say they believe the administration is under intense pressure from insurers and their allies to accommodate the business needs of insurers more than medical needs of patients. 'We have reason to fear that the external appeal regulations in particular won't be very consumer friendly,' said Stephen Finan, Senior Director of Policy for the American Cancer Society Action Network.

Representatives of several other consumer and patients' rights organizations, including Consumers Union, the National Partnership for Women and Families, and the American Diabetes Association, wrote in late January 2011 to officials in the Departments of Labor and Health and Human Services, pleading with them to 'stand firm for consumers' in rejecting several of the insurance industry's demands. They expressed concern that the final regulations would allow insurers to stack the decks against patients by allowing health plans to deem a second-level internal appeal of a denial as meeting the requirement for an independent external appeal. They're also worried that health plans will not be required to provide clear and understandable information to policyholders about their denial decisions, that the plans will not provide adequate translation of written communications into other languages (insurers are claiming this would be too burdensome), and that they will be able to take as long as seventy-two hours (instead of the recommended twenty-four) to decide an urgent appeal. The consumer advocates, most of whom, not so long ago, were applauding the Democrats for getting reform enacted, even if it fell short of their original goals, are becoming increasingly discouraged, partly because there are so many more lobbyists for the insurers than for consumers.

In April, insurers and several of their business allies announced the formation of the Choice and Competition Coalition (CCC) to influence the implementation of health care reform law at the state level. According to published reports, the CCC's membership includes America's Health Insurance Plans (AHIP), the US Chamber of Commerce, the Pharmaceutical Research and Manufacturers of America, and the National Association of Health Underwriters, which represents agents and brokers. The CCC reportedly will focus initially on the online health insurance marketplaces (the 'exchanges' that each state must set up by 2014). The group is expected to advocate for exchanges that allow any willing insurer to participate.

The reform law gives states wide latitude in how they operate their exchanges. When the California exchange is up and running in 2014, it will vet the insurers' benefit plans and offer only those it deems to be of value to consumers. Utah, on the other hand, established an exchange before the reform law was enacted, and insurers like it much better than what California is proposing. That's because the Utah exchange allows insurers to post all their benefit plans, even the ones with such limited benefits and high deductibles that many people who buy them are not adequately protected. Limited-benefit plans with high deductibles are especially profitable for insurers because they rarely have to pay out much in claims. The CCC is expected to be actively involved, operating, in many regards, like other front groups that insurers and other corporations have funded in years past.

What happens now?

The 2010 mid-term elections saw more money spent on campaigns than any non-presidential election in US history. In aggregate, between the spending of the two political parties, the candidates themselves, and outside groups, the election cost $4 billion.[14] The Supreme Court had ruled in January 2010 that the political contributions of US corporations could not be legally limited. Any company, lobbying group, or industry can give as much money as they desire to a candidate. And when these groups route their contributions through not-for-profit entities, a legal loophole allows them to remain anonymous. The ruling makes it possible for anyone with the available funds to spend them secretly on any political campaign they choose, saturating the airwaves with advertisements, paying canvassers to go door-to-door, funding phone banks, paying the postage on political mailers – virtually any activity in support of their candidate.

The Supreme Court's ruling gave rise to new political action committees – commonly known as 'super PACs' – whose fundraising capabilities are virtually unlimited. The best funded of them, according to the Center for Responsive Politics, was American Crossroads, a group led by Karl Rove, former top aide to President George W. Bush, and other prominent conservatives. American Crossroads spent $21.6 million by itself, accounting for 'one-third of all spending by super PACs this election … And American Crossroads itself nearly spent as much as all liberal-aligned super PACs combined.'[15]

The Center for Responsive Politics further reported in November 2010 that conservative-oriented super-PACs spent $34.7 million on the election. *U.S. News and World Report* put the figure at $39 million. Super-PACs were a powerful force in the election, but they weren't always successful. Democratic Senators Michael Bennet of Colorado and Harry Reid of Nevada were the primary targets of conservative groups, yet both won re-election. In all, American Crossroads and others spent almost $10 million in support of Bennet's and Reid's opponents.

In an October story in *The Washington Post*, the Federal Election Commission disclosed that the US Chamber of Commerce – a lobbying group representing large employers – had spent more than $10 million in one week in support of thirty-one Republican Congressional candidates (Eggen 2010). In all, the Chamber spent $33 million. Only American Crossroads spent more.[16] With the restrictions on their spending removed and their anonymity assured, industries funneled staggering amounts of money through their front groups to business-friendly, conservative candidates. And the mid-term elections ushered in a Republican majority in the House of Representatives and diminished the Democratic majority in the Senate.

The war between the states and the federal government

In all likelihood, the health care law as written represents the high-water mark for reform in the United States. Any changes that happen at the national level over the next several years are more likely to diminish the law's reach and impact than increase them. But, regardless of what happens at the federal level, the battle for the future of American health care in the United States will be waged in the states themselves, where the law has to be implemented.

A few examples:

In Idaho, lawmakers introduced a bill this year that would apply the late-eighteenth-century doctrine of nullification, based on some writings of Thomas Jefferson, asserting that states should be allowed their own interpretation of what is constitutional. Although Idaho's Attorney General wrote that nullification itself was unconstitutional – and most legal scholars agree with him – the bill was still introduced. And at least nine other states were also giving nullification serious consideration.[17]

Several states are asking for relief from the provision in the law that requires insurers' medical-loss ratio to stay above 80. Regulators in those states, including Florida, Kentucky, Iowa, and Kansas, fear that insurers may pull out of their markets rather than be compelled to give policyholders a rebate.[18]

More than half the states have filed lawsuits challenging the constitutionality of the reform law, in particular the individual mandate provision supported by insurers. The lawsuits assert that the law's tax penalty that would be levied on most people who do not buy health insurance sets a precedent that 'would imperil individual liberty, render Congress's other enumerated powers superfluous, and allow Congress to usurp the general police power reserved to the states.' The constitutionality of the law likely will be settled later this year or next by the US Supreme Court.[19]

An 'opt-out' provision that was written into the law, taking effect beginning in 2017, will allow states to request exemptions from certain requirements. In order to opt out, a state must provide coverage that is, at minimum, as comprehensive as the federal law and as affordable to consumers. The opt-out provision's author, Democrat Ron Wyden of Oregon, is now co-sponsoring a measure, along with Republican Scott Brown of Massachusetts, that would move the opt-out date up three years, to 2014. Proof of comprehensiveness and affordability should not prove difficult in Massachusetts. The state's coverage program, called Commonwealth Connector, was the template on which the federal law was fashioned. As of spring 2009 in Massachusetts, more than 97 percent of the population had health coverage (Trapp 2010).

South Carolina's Republican US Senator Lindsey Graham and Governor Nikki Haley are also working to opt out. 'I'm confident that, if given the chance, a large number of states would opt out of the provisions regarding the individual mandate,' Senator Lindsay Graham said. 'As more states opt out, it will have the effect of repealing and replacing Obamacare' (Eggen 2010). Graham and Haley claimed that the law would cost South Carolina $3.2 billion over ten years. S.C. Fair Share, a consumer advocacy group in South Carolina, claims that while the law will require $470 million in additional money from the state for Medicaid costs, the matching federal money will total almost $11 billion (Eggen 2010).

As the nominee to run the South Carolina Medicaid agency is being reviewed by a state committee, the only seat that remains vacant is the one allotted for a consumer advocate. Blue Cross Blue Shield of South Carolina has a seat, one that it lobbied assiduously to get. There is speculation in South Carolina and Florida that Blue Cross will take over the administration of Medicaid (Dudley 2011).

Florida Governor Rick Scott, a Republican and former CEO of a health care company, was expected to sign into law two bills that will effectively turn over 3 million Medicaid participants to the care of privately run, for-profit HMOs by 2012. The state is currently piloting a sweeping program designed to judge the viability of such a plan. Health professionals in the state worry that any savings achieved by the program will come at the cost of care.[20] Florida's new law would replace the fee-for-service system of reimbursement for doctors and pharmacies in favor of one that requires patients to enroll in an HMO or similar type of managed care plan. Managed care companies would be paid a set amount for each patient, and their profit would be based on how they manage their costs against that payment. A vascular surgeon was quoted in *The Washington Post*, saying, 'I just don't understand why Florida is pursuing a failing model' (Aizenman 2011).

In many other states, the area of contention in 2011 has been the state health insurance exchanges. In North Carolina, consumer and patient advocates were dealt a setback when the legislature passed a bill establishing the exchange that was drafted, at least in part, by Blue Cross Blue Shield of North Carolina. The bill gives the insurer a permanent seat on the exchange's board of directors. Several states are collaborating to establish multi-state 'compacts.' A compact, if approved by Congress, would allow the member states to introduce legislation that would supersede federal law. Consumer groups generally oppose compacts. They worry that it would render the federal reform law ineffectual.

In Vermont, arguably the country's most liberal state, Governor Shumlin has signed a bill into law that would establish a single-payer system, setting up a panel that will draft a proposal for universal coverage, called Green Mountain Care, available in 2017. Blue Cross Blue Shield of Vermont did not actively oppose the measure. The insurer would be a leading contender to administer the system, at least in part.

Vermonters are not the only supporters of a single-payer system. Lawmakers in California passed a single-payer bill twice during the administration of former Governor Arnold Schwarzenegger. Schwarzenegger vetoed both bills. Single-payer advocates in California are now at work on a different political strategy to move the idea forward. They believe that, if a single-payer type of system ever becomes reality in the United States, it will begin at the state level.

Lawmakers in Maine, in contrast, have proposed allowing state residents looking for coverage that does not come through an employer to shop in any other state in New England except Vermont.[21] Many of the bill's provisions, however, conflict with the federal law, such as the cap on how much older (and more expensive) participants can be charged for coverage. The Maine law will set it at five times the amount charged to a younger person. The federal requirement, which goes into effect in 2014, caps it at three times.

All of this activity in the states, and the numerous efforts in Washington to change or repeal parts or all of the new federal law, make it clear that the Affordable Care Act was not the final word on reform in the United States. Rather, it is better to think of the law as the end of the beginning of reform. It is also important to keep in mind that powerful special interests profiting from the *status quo* will continue to work behind the scenes, using the techniques of public relations to influence the public's perceptions and the drafting of the laws by which they will be compelled to live.

Manipulation of public opinion, the decline of mainstream journalism and the growth of corporate power

Alex Jones, director of Harvard University's Shorenstein Center on Press, Politics, and Public Policy, contends that American journalism is under assault. In his book *Losing the News*, he wrote: 'The profit squeeze has wreaked havoc on newsrooms and especially decimated the Washington-based press corps covering government on behalf of citizens back home' (Jones 2009). The number of credible news organizations in the United States, particularly newspapers, is declining. At the same time, the number of people, the amount of power, and the level of funding behind PR efforts are greater than ever, and are increasing. Americans are confronted daily – even hourly – with the daunting and growing challenge of deciphering truth from spin. With cutbacks in newsrooms, there are fewer reporters covering the health insurance industry than in years past, and those who are left are often so busy that they have little time to probe. Spin, however, remains plentiful and free.

This concept is similar to that of health care being accessible only to those with the resources to pay what the market demands. 'We may be headed for a world in which there is as yawning a disparity in accurate knowledge as there is in wealth,' Jones wrote. 'The elite will be deeply informed, and there will be a huge difference between what they know and what most other Americans know. We could be heading for a well-informed class at the top and a broad populace awash in opinion, spin, and propaganda' (Jones 2009: 21).

In the 1950s and 1960s, most major American cities had at least two daily newspapers, with morning and afternoon editions. As the pace of the news cycle increased and the influence of television grew, afternoon papers gradually shifted to a morning schedule or folded altogether, leaving late-day updates to broadcast media. Those major newspapers in major cities are rarer today. The 'iron core of information,' as Jones describes it, comes primarily from traditional news organizations, which provide 'accountability news' at the local, national, and international level. 'Traditional journalists have long believed that this form of fact-based accountability news is the essential food supply of democracy, and that without enough of this healthy nourishment, democracy will weaken, sicken, or even fail' (Jones 2009: 2–3).

'The Reconstruction of American Journalism,' a report published in the *Columbia Journalism Review* (CJR) in October 2009, stated:

> Newspapers and television news are not going to vanish in the foreseeable future, despite frequent predictions of their imminent extinction. But they will play diminished roles in an emerging and still rapidly changing world of digital journalism, in which the means of news reporting are being re-invented, the character of news is being reconstructed, and

reporting is being distributed across a greater number and variety of news organizations, new and old.

(Downie and Schudson 2009)

The *CJR* report explained the risks of the current trend:

What is under threat is independent reporting that provides information, investigation, analysis, and community knowledge, particularly in the coverage of local affairs … It may not be essential to save any particular news medium, including printed newspapers. What is paramount is preserving independent, original, credible reporting, whether or not it is popular or profitable, and regardless of the medium in which it appears.

(Downie and Schudson 2009: 11–12)

Efforts to manipulate opinion have grown increasingly pervasive over the past twenty years, in concert with the waning of traditional journalism in the United States. And with less access to credible information, Americans are more easily manipulated. The fate of reform, the nature of debate, and perhaps even the fate of democracy in the United States may be determined by the ability of Americans to find reliable information and to see through spin from the special interests invested in the outcome.

Notes

1 Karen Davis, PhD, Cathy Schoen, MS, and Kristof Stremikis, MPP, *Mirror, Mirror on the Wall: How the Performance of the U.S. Health Care System Compares Internationally, 2010 Update*, Commonwealth Fund, June 2010.
2 Kaiser Family Foundation, *How Private Health Coverage Works: A Primer – 2008 Update*, April 2008.
3 Centers for Medicare and Medicaid Services, 'National Health Expenditures Historicals for 1960–2007', table 16, Centers for Medicare and Medicaid Services, U.S. Department of Health and Human Services. www.cms.hhs.gov/NationalHealth ExpendData/downloads/tables.pdf
4 Frank Luntz, 'The language of healthcare 2009'. http://wonkroom.thinkprogress. org/wp-content/uploads/2009/05/frank-luntz-the-language-of-healthcare-20091.pdf
5 Bill Adair and Angie Drobnic Holan, 'PolitiFact's Lie of the Year: "A government takeover of health care"', Politifact.com, December 16, 2010. www.politifact.com/ truth-o-meter/article/2010/dec/16/lie-year-government-takeover-health-care
6 *Ibid.*
7 Lindsay Renick Mayer, 'Insurers fight public health plan', Center for Responsive Politics, June 18, 2009. www.opensecrets.org/news/2009/06/insurers-fight-public-health-p.html
8 Public Campaign Action Fund, 'Insurance and HMOs spend nearly $700,000 per day to kill health care reform measures', Public Campaign Action Fund, September 15, 2009. www.campaignmoney.org/HMO_insurance_spend_to_kill_reform
9 Centers for Medicare and Medicaid Services, 'National Health Expenditures Historicals for 1960–2007', table 16, Centers for Medicare and Medicaid Services, U.S. Department of Health and Human Services. www.cms.hhs.gov/NationalHealth ExpendData/downloads/tables.pdf

10 John Sheils and Randy Haught, *The Cost and Coverage Impacts of a Public Plan: Alternative Design Options*, The Lewin Group, April 8, 2009.
11 Alan Fram, 'Top insurance lobbyist: August key in health drive', Associated Press, August 10, 2009.
12 Jesse Lee, 'Reality check: AHIP's "study" hard to take seriously', White House Blog, October 12, 2009.
13 U.S. Department of Labor, Employee Benefits Security Administration, *The Affordable Care Act: Protecting Consumers and Putting Patients Back in Charge of Their Care*, July 22, 2010.
14 Danielle Kurtzleben, '2010 set campaign spending records', *U.S. News & World Report*, January 7, 2011.
15 Michael Beckel, 'Led by Karl Rove-linked groups, "Super PACs" and nonprofits significantly aid GOP in election 2010', Center for Responsive Politics, November 5, 2010. www.opensecrets.org/news/2010/11/led-by-karl-rove-linked-groups-nonp.html
16 Danielle Kurtzleben, '2010 set campaign spending records', U.S. News & World Report, January 7, 2011.
17 Associated Press, 'GOP dusts off 1700s doctrine. Latest volley against health care reform based on Jefferson's "nullification"', *Grand Rapids Press*, January 27, 2011.
18 Julie Appleby, 'States seek to soften rule on insurers' profits, millions of dollars in consumer rebates at stake', *Kaiser Health News*, May 16, 2011.
19 Greg Bluestein, 'States ask US court to overturn health overhaul', Associated Press, May 5, 2011.
20 Kelli Kennedy and Brent Kallestad, 'Florida Senate passes historic Medicaid overhaul', Associated Press, May 6, 2011.
21 Kevin Miller, 'Maine Senate enacts sweeping partisan health insurance reform', May 16, 2011, http:/bangordailynews.com/2011/05/16/politics/maine-senate-enacts_health-insurance-overhaul/

References

Aizenman, N.C. (2011) 'Fla. test of privatizing Medicaid raises more questions', *The Washington Post*, May 12.
Begley, S. (2009) 'The five biggest lies in the health care debate', *Newsweek*, September 7.
Clinton, W.J. (2004) *My Life*, New York: Alfred A. Knopf.
Daschle, T. (2008) *Critical: What We Can Do About the Health-Care Crisis*, New York: Thomas Dunne Books.
DeNavas-Watt, C., Proctor, B.D. and Smith, J.C. (2010) *Income, Poverty and Health Insurance Coverage in the United States: 2009*, U.S. Census Bureau, Current Population Reports, p60–238, Washington, D.C.: U.S. Government Printing Office. www.census.gov/prod/2010pubs/p60-238.pdf
Dionne Jr, E.J. (2003) 'Ted and Hillary's health care split', *The Washington Post*, June 24.
Downie, L. and Schudson, M. (2009) 'The reconstruction of American journalism', *Columbia Journalism Review*, October 19.
Dudley, R. (2011) 'S.C. lays health exchange groundwork. Insurer's inclusion on board leads to advocates' concerns', *Charleston Post and Courier*, May 21.
Eggen, D. (2010) 'U.S. Chamber puts millions into GOP ads', *The Washington Post*, October 29.
Good, C. (2009) 'The Tea Party movement: who's in charge?' *The Atlantic*, April 13.
Hacker, J.S. (2008) 'The case for public plan choice in national health reform: key cost control and quality coverage', *Institute for America's Future*, December 16. www.law.berkeley.edu/files/Hacker-PublicPlan-Final109.pdf

Henderson, E.L. (1949) 'Statement on Truman Health Plan', *JAMA*, 140(1): 114–19.

Hilzenrath, D. (2009) 'Insurer-owned consulting firm often cited in health debate', *The Washington Post*, July 23.

Helfand, D. (2010) 'Anthem Blue Cross dramatically raising rates for Californians with individual health policies', *Los Angeles Times*, February 4.

Jones, A.S. (2009) *Losing the News*, Oxford: Oxford University Press.

Kmietowicz, Z. and Ferriman, A. (2002) 'Pro-tobacco writer admits he should have declared an interest', *British Medical Journal*, 324: 257.1.

Murray, S. and Montgomery, L. (2009) 'Prognosis improves for public insurance', *The Washington Post*, October 24.

PR Newswire (1992) 'Humana chairman sees opportunity and challenge in health care reform', *PR Newswire*, November 13.

Quadagno, J. (2005) *One Nation Uninsured: Why the U.S. Has No National Health Insurance*, Oxford: Oxford University Press.

Skocpol, T. (1995) 'The demise of the Clinton plan', *Health Affairs*, Spring: 66–85.

Starr, P. (1982) *The Social Transformation of American Medicine*, New York: Basic Books.

Stone, P.H. (1994) 'Lost cause', *National Journal*, September.

Terhune, C. and Epstein, K. (2009) 'The health insurers have already won', *Business Week*, August 6.

Trapp, D. (2010) 'Cost increases tied to market power's impact on payment: Mass. Study', *American Medical News*, February 22. www.ama-assn.org/amednews/2010/02/22/gvsc0222.htm.

WHO (2000) *World Health Report 2000. Health Systems: Improving Performance*, Geneva: World Health Organization.

Wynn, P. (1996) 'What the For-Profit Trend in Health Care Really Means', *Managed Care*, June.

2   The break-up of the NHS: implications for information systems[1]

Allyson Pollock and David Price

Introduction

Tax funded universal health systems are characterised by administrative functions that focus on needs assessment and resource allocation across geographic populations so as to ensure comprehensive coverage that is country and system-wide. This is because in universal systems, financial risk is pooled at government level. In market systems, however, financial risks are allocated (spread) across different parts of the system through market contracting. Administrative functions in these systems focus on risk pricing and segmentation among providers, members or enrollees. Using the example of the English National Health Service (NHS), we argue that the information systems required to enable risk segmentation are different from those underpinning comprehensive care. Administration is non-geographic in market bureaucracies and geographic in comprehensive systems. This leads to a shift in information requirements that poses difficulties for resource allocation and service planning, and therefore for universalist goals.

Since 1948, the NHS has assumed the responsibility for the risks and costs of health care for all citizens. However, a succession of statutory changes dating back to 1990, and culminating in the Health and Social Care Act 2012 (House of Commons 2012), have increasingly undermined this national responsibility. When the latest Act comes into effect, risks and costs will be spread among government funders, local authorities, insurers, providers, the public and, ultimately, patients.

The Act introduces new structures taken from the American health maintenance organisation (HMO) industry, in which commercial organisations insure and provide care for a selected membership rather than geographic populations (Pollock and Price 2011). The introduction of these structures to the NHS is accompanied by a major overhaul of administrative structures involving the substitution of market for public bureaucracies. The new market bureaucracies will give discretion to commissioners to define the scope of NHS services and, to some extent, to select the population for which they purchase care. They will also allow providers to select the publicly financed services for which they tender. Deregulation of this type facilitates the emergence of business strategies based on risk-selection.

Such was the strength of public opposition to the bill during its passage through parliament that, in April 2011, the prime minister suspended the legislative process for three months and instigated a special forum to hear and respond to public and professional concerns. However, in spite of 300 significant amendments by the government, criticism of the new Act continues. The government has now abolished the Minister's duty to provide comprehensive care throughout England, and created an independent body, the NHS Commissioning Board, to oversee commissioning. The fundamental concern is that abolition will result in a loss of the universal and comprehensive character of the NHS and pave the way for a switch from taxed-based to insurance-based financing and user charges (Pollock and Price 2011).

In this chapter, we focus on the new administrative bureaucracy that is necessary to support market reform of this type. We show that information is key to our understanding, specifically the change in the unit of analysis associated with a shift in responsibility from area-based populations to membership-based systems akin to insurance pools. This analytical change also facilitates a transfer of risk from government to patients.

Market bureaucracies

For the past twenty-five years, in common with many health systems, NHS reform has been profoundly influenced by market theory (Walsh 1995; NHS 2000; Mossialos et al. 2002; Shen and Melnick 2004; Jamison et al. 2006; Boyle 2007; WHO 2008). Among the most widely pursued policies internationally are the substitution on economic grounds of competing, commercial providers for publicly administered government units, and the introduction or extension of competition among third-party payers and insurers of health care.

The introduction of these markets has implications for public health bureaucracies in terms of their control over the various components of health systems. Whilst the impact of markets on public health functions such as workforce planning and financial incentives has attracted considerable research (Rechel et al. 2009; WHO 2006; Reich et al. 2008; Reich and Takemi 2009), less attention has been given to their impact on population data. However, market systems require a different analytical framework from publicly integrated ones, and this in turn affects the data systems and the information used.

Tax funded universal health systems are characterised by administrative functions that focus on needs assessment and resource allocation across geographic populations and system-wide. This is because in universal systems financial risk is pooled at government level and the whole population must be comprehensively covered. The NHS is a prime example of the geographic focus that has grown up around a virtually monopolistic provider of health care and has encouraged extensive data collection and analysis on population health, health inequalities and access to health care by social class and ethnicity.

These are the data that the market analytic threatens. In market systems, financial risks are allocated across different parts of the system through market contracting, and there is no duty to provide services on a comprehensive basis or to collect data on a geographic basis. Instead, administrative functions in market systems focus on risk pricing and segmentation among providers, members or enrollees. In advocating market or 'strategic purchasing' as an important tool for improving health system cost efficiency, the authors of the World Health Report 2000 (WHO 2000) largely overlooked the implications of this different analysis for information.

The impact of markets on some public health functions is relatively well understood. For example, market-related, unmanaged outflows of health workers are known to damage health systems, undermine planning projections and erode the skills base, according to the World Health Organization (Rechel 2006). The workforce crisis among trained personnel in resource-poor countries has recently been recognised as an issue in international aid (WHO 2006; Reich et al. 2008; Reich and Takemi 2009). Following the *World Health Report 2006*, which estimated a staffing shortfall of 4 million in developing countries, the first global forum on workforce issues was held in Kampala in 2008.

Another example is the lack of routine data in marketised health systems, which have underdeveloped, population-based information systems because public authorities do not have planning powers or resources to justify their collection (Pollock and Rice 1997), or because large proportions of the population are not covered. The efficiency of planning systems depends to a large extent on routine data collection and the power of public bodies to require data returns from providers. Loss of this capacity can be seen very directly in the UK's long-term sector, where, in 1991, the private sector and local authorities were allowed to pass risks back from the NHS to the public via new eligibility criteria involving a means test. The planning, resourcing and provision of care of older people to this day is left to the market, and it is now impossible to assess on a population basis the scale and distribution of resources devoted to the various elements of care, because data that would allow these assessments are no longer available.

The effect of privatisation on data availability for long-term care suggests a wider question about the role data can play when governments seek to withdraw from universal policies. In long-term care, planning data did not merely cease to be available; they were no longer officially needed because the government had largely relinquished responsibility and thus financial risk for care. Normative change of this sort is undoubtedly assisted by absence of evidence of unmet need and hardship.

The shift from integrated public to market health care systems requires innovations in the identification of risk, which in turn change the basis of health information. For example, markets require incorporation of providers so that risk can be allocated through commercial contracting; they involve changes to revenue and capital accounting so that commercial loans can be substituted for government grants; they typically include revised reimbursement mechanisms based on price signals, in which case- or activity-based payments to providers are substituted for block grants (Gaffney et al. 1999a–c); and, to facilitate 'consumer choice' or incentivise providers, they are commonly associated with new performance management frameworks with a focus on firms or providers rather than whole populations living in contiguous areas (Jacobson et al. 2003; Bottle et al. 2011).

How the integrated approach of risk-pooling is achieved in a universal public bureaucracy

Throughout most of its sixty-three-year existence, the NHS has had a duty to employ administrative structures that promote equity and redistribution through resource allocation, service planning and needs assessment. The issue of how government deals with catastrophic risks and costs on behalf of its citizens was the normative problem addressed by the introduction of the welfare state in the UK, and the systems of benefits that underpinned it (Timmins 2001). Accordingly, the structures of the NHS were originally based on contiguous or seamless geographic tiers of administration designed to ensure universal coverage. Service providers were directly administered and integrated into the organisation with responsibility for meeting needs and planning services. There was no billing, invoicing or contracting and, crucially, no selection or denial of care on the basis of place of residence or ability to pay. Instead, resource-allocation methods and service planning dealt with universal populations. The denominator was always all the citizens living within a geographic area drawn from census or census estimates; the numerators comprised the subgroups of specific interest, which always related back to the whole population. These methods proved to be highly efficient, and the NHS was one of the lowest-cost universal systems in the world (Pollock 2005).

The risk-allocation approach of a market

Market and business strategies focus on individuals or groups of individuals as customers or members of insurance pools. The denominators here are members or enrollees, a provider's customer list, or an insurer's list of potential claimants. Under the new bill, it will be patient registrations belonging to the lists of general practitioners (family doctors). To maximise income and profit, market actors must now engage in complicated risk-selection strategies that enable them to avoid contracting for high-risk patients and treatments or for markets with low profitability. Examples of risk-selection methods include the differential premiums charged by insurance companies, or the range of tiered benefit plans offered to consumers: a minimum package, or higher benefits price with risk sharing or co-insurance, time limits on care, or an annual cap on attendances, for example. Risks are identified in market contracts that function as the legal means by which risks are allocated and paid for. There is little or no empirical verification of the cost-efficiency claims made for market structures (Perrot 2004; Loevinsohn and Harding 2005; Liu et al. 2007) whilst their effect on equity is largely unevaluated (Liu et al. 2008; Peters et al. 2009).

The risk shift

Under the NHS Act, risk analyses will become central to both the public and private side of contracting. Private firms require services and patient lists to be unbundled so that they have the ability to select on commercial grounds. Meanwhile, in an attempt to counter risk-selection of this type, or its consequences, the government will seek to risk-adjust provider incentives (for example, through adjustments to diagnosis-related group reimbursement) or to equalise risk among different payer organisations with disparate, and not necessarily equally high-risk, memberships (Van de Ven et al. 2003; Van de Ven 2011).

A shift to market bureaucracies requires a change in the information that underpins the methods for funding and financing. In the first three of five examples, we show how the information requirement changes and, in so doing, the unit of analysis changes from comprehensive area-based populations to members or providers that do not provide comprehensive care to all. In the fourth and fifth examples we show the implications of this change in information for performance measurement and comparisons of health systems.

1. Changes in the system of resource allocation: from areas to members

The current system of resource allocation

Since 1948, area-based funding has been the method of allocating resources across England for the NHS. Area-based formulae have been used since the 1970s to distribute resources fairly among the 'local populations', 'catchments' or 'resident populations' of primary care trusts (PCTs):

> Primary care trusts (PCTs) are responsible for funding NHS hospitals, GPs and other health care services for their local populations.

> The Government, through the Department of Health, provides the money to all of the 151 PCTs across the country to fund these health services.

> The Department sets PCTs' budgets in advance, mainly on the basis of a formula to calculate each PCT's fair share of the total available budget for England.

In 2011–12, the total health budget for PCTs was £89 billion and the Department has to find a way for allocating this between PCTs in a fair way.

(Department of Health 2011a)

Since its inception, the NHS has been based on the principle of equal access for equal need. This principle is embodied in two longstanding objectives for resource allocation from the centre to local health services:

- To distribute resources based on the relative need of each area for health services. Currently, this objective is to enable PCTs to commission the same levels of health services for populations with similar needs;
- In addition, to contribute to the reduction in avoidable health inequalities.

(Department of Health 2011b)

The resource allocation formulae devised to meet these objectives include: the age profile of the population (localities with more elderly populations have higher needs, all else being equal); additional need over and above that relating to age (localities with less healthy populations and higher levels of deprivation have higher needs, all else being equal); and unavoidable geographic differences in the cost of providing services – the market forces factor (it costs more to provide the same level of services in high-cost areas such as London and the south-east). The formulae have been the subject of revision over many decades.

How the resource-allocation system will change under the Act

Under the Health and Social Care Act 2012, the Secretary of State's principal duty remains unchanged, and under Clause 10(2) the duty to 'arrange for the provision of services to such extent as it considers necessary … to meet … reasonable requirements' (House of Commons 2012) is transferred to commissioning groups. Commissioning groups, however, will not be contiguous, geographic, area-based administrative structures, they will be membership organisations.

Moreover, the Department of Health Memorandum to the Delegated Powers and Regulatory Reform Committee (Department of Health 2011c: paras 53 and 57) states that the intention of Clauses 10 and 11 is to allow commissioning groups discretion with respect to the selection of patients and services, and that this discretion will be limited by regulation.

Thus responsibility for provision will no longer be to all persons in an area, but only to 'persons for whom it [the clinical commissioning group, CCG] has responsibility' (House of Commons 2012); nor will it involve purchasing all services deemed part of a comprehensive health system.

The Act and the new structures have been anticipated for quite some time. For the past few years, behind the scenes the civil service has been at work to effect that transformation. In 2010, well in advance of the legislation, the Secretary of State instructed the Advisory Committee on Resource Allocation to switch from 2013 from PCT- and area-based populations to GP registrations in deriving its new formulae (Department of Health 2010a). This is in recognition of the fact that CCGs will not have the same geographic basis as PCTs because they are able to include patients registered with GP practices anywhere in England. They are only required to have 'a sufficient geographic focus to be able to take responsibility for agreeing and monitoring contracts for locality-based services (such as urgent care services), to have responsibility for commissioning services for people who are not registered with a GP practice, and to commission services jointly with local authorities' (Department of Health 2010b: 29). However, 'sufficient geographic focus' is not otherwise defined.

'Fair allocation' objectives need to be embodied in the new NHS system, but this is made almost impossible by the loss of responsibility for a defined geographic population. It is unclear, for example, if and how a measure such as disability-free life expectancy (DFLE) could be derived for CCGs, given their irregular, non-geographic, overlapping mosaic of footprints.

Since CCGs will no longer be geographically focused, the loss of area-based population responsibilities has serious implications for the stability and accuracy of measurements of need and for the equity of resource allocation and funding. In the absence of area-based planning information, CCGs will be able to manage their risks and costs in different ways.

2. Capital planning protocols – from area-based needs to provider's affordability under resource accounting and the private finance initiative

From capital grants to debts and private finance

The problems of fairness of funding highlighted in the Act are not new to the NHS. They have already been played out in capital allocations for new hospitals under the Private Finance Initiative (PFI), a policy introduced in 1991 according to which new capital is distributed among hospitals on the basis of provider finances rather than area needs criteria. Before PFI, NHS capital budgets were allocated as block grants on the basis of need and regional development plans. Financial reforms in 1990 effectively transformed grants into loans that local service providers were responsible for repaying to the Treasury. PFI exploited this development by transforming debts to the Treasury into debts to private consortiums, with local service providers still responsible for repayment. The result was that budgetary allocations for new building were no longer awarded to areas on behalf of the whole population on the basis of need, but were given to providers to finance loan repayment (Gaffney et al. 1999a–c) on the basis of what commissioners thought they could afford to pay from their revenue budgets.

NHS hospitals award PFI contracts to the private sector to design, build, finance and operate new facilities. Because investment and operating costs are paid for out of hospital operating budgets, before its introduction PFI required the creation of a special revenue stream that could be directed to pay for capital. This in turn required the government to change its financing method for hospital building from capital grants to loans, and it required hospitals and services to put their accounting on a commercial basis in order to reflect the new element of capital charging in their financial management.

Shifting the risk

Crucially, the impact of PFI was to shift risk of capital budgets from national and regional level to local providers, making them responsible for the affordability of capital. This type of risk devolution impairs the geographic focus underpinning service planning because it makes providers' debts and debt servicing a higher priority than funding capital health care needs (Gaffney et al. 1999a). In early PFIs, planning took place outside public health, as teams of management consultants were brought in to model bed closures using implausible productivity targets in order that the clinical budget could be redirected to pay for capital at the expense of clinical care. Thus PFI planning and allocations for capital turn on the question of what a hospital can afford to pay (or rather borrow), not on the health care needs of a geographic population for capital (Gaffney and Pollock 1999; Gaffney et al. 1999a–c).

PFI is also based on a form of revenue unbundling necessary for risk allocation. A typical PFI contract involves separating out revenue streams for capital, maintenance and some ancillary services in order that risks can be transferred or allocated in different proportions and to different parties. This is because the PFI contract involves specifying and pricing risks that the private sector is paid to undertake instead of the public sector.

PFI is a good example of the new market analytic at work. It shows how the information requirements changed from capital needs to the affordability of debt repayment at provider level and displaced the role of area-based needs data in capital allocation. It also highlights difficulties in provider-level calculations of cost efficiency arising from the arbitrary or contentious nature of risk pricing and the way in which risk was shifted.

3. Commissioning and contracting with private providers: the case of the ISTC

Risk segmentation through patient selection

The UK's £4 billion independent sector treatment centre (ISTC) programme provides a third example of how a non-comprehensive provider focus erodes area-based population data, in this case as a result of selection bias in the allocation of patients to, and non-recording of, data by the commercial sector.

In 2000, the UK government announced a plan to contract out elective surgery under the ISTC programme (Pollock and Kirkwood 2009). The opportunity to purchase care from the commercial sector under this scheme represented a major departure from the original model of the NHS as virtual monopoly provider of publicly financed hospital services. In order to facilitate commercial participation, two important risk-management measures were adopted. In the first place, elective surgery was unbundled (or cases differentiated according to criteria of complexity such as age and co-morbidity) so that more complex and potentially higher-cost cases could be left with NHS facilities, and commercial providers could concentrate on high-volume, low-risk operations. The separation was achieved by making it mandatory to risk-select patients through treatment protocols. Secondly, demand risk was retained by the state via the adoption of 'take-or-pay' contracts, according to which contractors were to be paid for a set number of operations whether or not this number of patients actually materialised.

Loss of population data

With providers not bound by the same data-collection duties as the NHS, and standards of collection largely unmonitored or poor, the intrusion of risk-selection was to have a profound effect on public health data. Mason and colleagues (Mason et al. 2010) at the University of York have shown that ISTCs do not collect good, timely data, and that such data as are collected show that ISTCs recruit and select from a healthier patient population. This selection will, of course, affect hospital league tables and general performance data (see below). It also undermines routine data collection, which ceases to be comprehensive.

Evaluation of the ISTC programme was itself a victim of these new weaknesses, as the data were not available to carry out a reliable assessment (Pollock and Kirkwood 2009). Strikingly, evaluation in Scotland was carried out by the management consultants who had helped the government set up the programme.

This example shows that data collection is fundamentally affected when patient selection is allowed. In the first place, data integrity and continuity are undermined. Secondly, aggregate output or outcome data cease to have meaning because they reflect risk-selection, not relative performance.

4. How international comparisons of health system performance obscure risk-selection and ignore differences in population – the case of Kaiser Permanente

It is possible to see risk-selection play out in comparisons of health system performance both at provider level and internationally. In 2002, Richard Feachem and colleagues (Feachem et al. 2002) published a paper purporting to compare the cost efficiency of the NHS with that of Kaiser Permanente, an American HMO. In fact it illustrates the way in which risk-selection undermines health system comparison. HMOs are premised on patient and service selection, they combine insurer and provider functions, and their populations comprise members or enrollees. The populations are unstable due to high enrolment and disenrolment rates; coverage is not universal, nor does it serve contiguous areas; and risk-selection is rife. Accordingly, aggregate performance data will reflect relative success in selection, not relative success in attaining comprehensive cover within areas, which is the goal of the NHS.

Health system comparison has become an important tool in the political management of market reform. Frequently used to evaluate performance among systems at different stages of marketisation (Nolte et al. 2005), international comparisons are increasingly used to assess the relative effectiveness of different structural elements from a cost-containment perspective. Comparisons of this type are fraught with methodological difficulties because health care systems can be more or less selective. Comparisons between universal and non-universal systems are deeply problematical because like is not being compared with like.

Measurement and reporting issues can also confound results because of differences in the definition of health spending, under-reporting and over-reporting, and variation in methods for measuring the size of the informal sector. Price comparison is also problematic. Prices can be compared by converting into US dollar equivalents using current exchange rates, or by estimating 'purchasing power parity' (PPP), also referred to as the 'international dollar rate'. PPPs involve contestable assumptions about market prices and the costs they reflect.

These problems were apparent in the paper by Feachem and colleagues published in the *British Medical Journal* in 2002, shortly after the *NHS Plan* (NHS 2000) announced the introduction of the provider market (Feachem et al. 2002). The paper's authors purported to show that Kaiser Permanente was more cost-efficient than the NHS, and that risk-selection and other problems of comparison had been taken into account. However, within a week of publication, the BMJ had 170 responses mostly critical of data, methods and assumptions (Talbot-Smith et al. 2004).

Crucially, the populations served by Kaiser and the NHS are very different, and so too are the range of benefits. Whereas the NHS provides universal, comprehensive cover to all citizens in the UK, around 60 million people, largely free of charge, Kaiser recruits healthier, wealthier and younger patients as members of plans with restricted benefits and numerous additional charges, and does not provide comprehensive care (Talbot-Smith et al. 2004). No amount of risk adjustment can adjust for these differences; Kaiser's population can never be risk-adjusted to become like the NHS, as it was never designed to be comprehensive.

This case study shows a deliberate attempt to promote as more efficient a system in which competing insurers and providers can optimise their risks by selection. However, the more an insurer and provider can risk-select, the more cost efficient it is likely to appear. In fact, the paper rested on erroneous methodology and false claims.

5. How hospital league tables engender risk-selection

The switch to providers and members as part of risk-selection strategies of market-oriented systems is played out in performance measures locally. Performance league tables, widely promoted as a means of privatising provision (Rechel et al. 2009), also reflect a shift from universality to risk individualisation by substituting provider-based performance for measures of access and equity at area level. They are products of economic theory that predicts markets will work imperfectly in circumstances where purchasers do not have full information. This problem, known among economists as 'information asymmetry' (Arrow 1963), is particularly acute in health care, where providers know far more than purchasers and are easily able to trade off cost against quality, because the latter is so difficult to measure. League tables are intended to overcome this tendency by making comparisons of outcomes publicly available.

Hospital-based mortality rates are often favoured as the measure of hospital quality; the reality is that area-based mortality should be the focus. Jacobson et al. (2003) and, more recently, Bottle et al. (2011) have shown weaknesses in hospital mortality league tables. Among the problems identified are:

- quality of data and coding the numerator problem of deaths – patients may die on their way to hospital or because of delays in referral; some may die out of hospital; others may be admitted but discharged and then readmitted to other hospitals before death, and here the response is to apportion a death to all of the hospitals – the patient dies not once but several times over in several different hospitals
- denominator problems – the population is unstable and comprises those who can get access, but how are they counted – as admissions, first admissions or finished consultant episodes (FCEs), and which population do you count?
- case-mix adjustment – different hospitals have different mixes of patients and services
- institutional issues – small hospitals, poor quality and lack of data, coding, incompleteness of data, inability to adjust for institutional differences.

If they are to convey reliable information, league tables must at least adjust for differences in the risks present in different populations. However, risk-adjustment methodologies are often spurious, and involve unreliable data and complex modelling that conceals bias. In a landmark critique of hospital league tables in the *Journal of the Royal Statistical Society*, Goldstein and Spiegelhalter (1996: 389) conclude: 'No amount of fancy statistical footwork will overcome basic inadequacies in either the appropriateness or the integrity of the data collected.'

The journals are bursting with critiques of league tables, but public authorities are impervious to them, and use and publish them for marketing and recruitment purposes. A more profound problem arises when this type of data is used as the basis for pricing and cost comparisons, and to determine whether an NHS hospital goes into deficit and whether it stays open or closes. More recently, economists have tried to argue that hospital concentration and competition saves lives, based on erroneous assumptions and data of this type (Pollock et al. 2011). However, such performance league tables can discourage clinicians and providers from treating patients with high morbidity and high costs.

And yet the geographic population focus of a public health frame is far simpler. For many decades, public health has analysed variations in treatment, service use and access over time between and across populations, districts or PCTs and by social class. These data have been used to conduct sensible, detailed audits, confidential enquiries, surveys and investigations into the whole patient pathway, including referrals from and access to primary care.

Conclusion

It has long been recognised that health care planning and equitable resource allocation cannot be left to the invisible hand of the market. As Abel-Smith put it in 1976, markets mean that there is 'no single organization pledged to provide the best health service possible out of a limited budget' (Abel-Smith 1976: 154). The NHS was originally conceived as a non-market model in order to optimise resource use. However, our case studies show that a comprehensive service requires an administrative bureaucracy underpinned by information consistent with that function. Public bureaucracies are not destroyed overnight, but rather through a succession of technical incremental changes to the information systems that inform the systems for resource allocation, capital allocation, and coverage and provision. Where risk segmentation is the goal, then there is an interplay between information and resource-allocation systems that changes the data requirements in fundamental ways, so that the focus shifts from area-based populations to aggregates of individuals or enrollees for the purpose of risk management. This shift fundamentally affects the availability, production and analysis of area-based comprehensive data. Finally, once introduced, risk-based data can be used to undermine universal systems by allowing providers and commissioners to be selective about coverage and care. This switch in data systems is therefore both a cause and a consequence of market fragmentation, and enables the shift from national risk-pooling to risk-selection.

Central to all this is the unit of analysis. When the focus ceases to be comprehensive health care to the whole population living within an area, and becomes instead risk allocation to individuals, members, enrollees or providers, then universality is no longer attainable because the necessary data underpinning it are no longer available, and providers have the opportunity to risk-select. As we show in our examination of the latest NHS legislative proposals, this change of focus is a way of managing the normative transition from universality to selection (Pollock and Price 2011). That is why we have concluded that the information requirements that underpin risk-selection contribute to the abolition of the NHS as a universal system of health care.

Note

1 A version of this article originally appeared in *Michael Quarterly* 8 (2011): 460–75. Reproduced with kind permission.

References

Abel-Smith, B. (1976) *Value for Money in Health Services*, London: Heinemann.
Arrow, K.A. (1963) 'Uncertainty and the welfare economics of medical care', *American Economic Review*, 53(5): 941–73.
Bottle, A., Jarman, B. and Aylin, P. (2011) 'Strengths and weaknesses of hospital standardised mortality ratios', *BMJ*, 342: c7116.
Boyle, N. H. (2007) 'The case for private provision in the NHS', *Annals of the Royal College of Surgeons of England*, 89(4): 337–41.
Department of Health (2010a) *Advisory Committee on Resource Allocation: Summary of Recommendations*. www.dh.gov.uk/en/ManagingyourOrganization/Financeandplanning/Allocations/index.htm
——(2010b) *Equity and Excellence: Liberating the NHS*, Cm7881, London: Stationery Office. www.dh.gov.uk/en/Publicationsandstatistics/Publications/PublicationsPolicy AndGuidance/DH_117353
——(2011a) *Use of Information on the Number of People Registered with each GP Practice for NHS Allocations (Budgets)*. www.dh.gov.uk/en/Managingyourorganisation/Financea ndplanning/Allocations/DH_125268
——(2011b) *Resource Allocation: Weighted Capitation Formula*, 7th edn, London: Department of Health.
——(2011c) *Health and Social Care Bill 2011 Memorandum for the House of Lords Delegated Powers and Regulatory Reform Committee* (updated to reflect the Bill as introduced in the House of Lords).
Feachem, R.G.A., Sekhri, N.K. and White, K. (2002) 'Getting more for their dollar: a comparison of the NHS with California's Kaiser Permanente', *BMJ*, 324: 135–43.
Gaffney, D. and Pollock, A.M. (1999) 'Pump-priming the PFI: why are privately financed hospital schemes being subsidized?' *Public Money & Management*, 19: 55–62.
Gaffney, D., Pollock, A.M., Price, D. and Shaoul, J. (1999a) 'NHS capital expenditure and the private finance initiative – expansion or contraction?' *BMJ.*, 319: 48–51.
——(1999b) 'PFI in the NHS – is there an economic case?' *BMJ*, 319: 116–19.
——(1999c) 'The politics of the private finance initiative and the new NHS', *BMJ*, 319: 249–53.
Goldstein, H. and Spiegelhalter, D. J. (1996) 'League tables and their limitations: statistical issues in comparisons of institutional performance', *JRSS*, 159: 385–443.

House of Commons (2012) *Health and Social Care Act 2012*, London: HMSO.

Jacobson, B., Mindell, J. and McKee, M. (2003) 'Hospital mortality league tables', *BMJ*, 326: 777–78.

Jamison, D., Breman, J., Measham, A., Alleyne, G., Claeson, M., Evans, D., Jha, P., Mills, A. and Musgrove, P. (eds) (2006) *Disease Control Priorities in Developing Countries*, 2nd edn, Washington: The International Bank for Reconstruction and Development / The World Bank.

Liu, X., Hotchkiss, D.R. and Bose, S. (2008) 'The effectiveness of contracting-out primary health care services in developing countries: a review of the evidence', *Health Policy Plan*, 23(1): 1–13.

——(2007) 'The impact of contracting-out on health system performance: a conceptual framework', *Health Policy*, 82: 200–211.

Loevinsohn, B. and Harding, A. (2005) 'Buying results? Contracting for health service delivery in developing countries', *Lancet*, 366: 676–81.

Mason, A., Street, A. and Verzulli, R. (2010) 'Private sector treatment centres are treating less complex patients than the NHS', *JRSM*, 103: 322–31.

Mossialos, E., Dixon, A., Figueras, J. and Kutzin, J. (eds) (2002) *Funding Health Care: Options for Europe*, Maidenhead: Open University Press.

NHS (2000) *NHS Plan*, London: National Health Service.

Nolte, M., McKee, M. and Wait, S. (2005) 'Describing and evaluating health systems'. In A. Bowling and S. Ebrahim (eds) *Handbook of Health Research Methods*, Maidenhead: Open University Press.

Perrot, J. (2004) *The Role of Contracting in Improving Health Systems Performance Discussion Paper No. 1*, Geneva: World Health Organization.

Peters, D., El-Saharty, S., Siadat, B., Janovsky, K. and Vujicic, M. (eds) (2009) *Improving Healthservice Delivery in Developing Countries: From Evidence to Action*, Washington, DC: World Bank.

Pollock, A.M. (2005) *NHS plc*. London: Verso.

Pollock, A.M. and Kirkwood, G. (2009) 'Independent sector treatment centres: learning from a Scottish case study', *BMJ*, 338: b1421.

Pollock, A.M. and Price, D. (2011) 'How the Secretary of State for Health proposes to abolish the NHS in England', *BMJ*, 342: d1695.

Pollock, A.M. and Rice, D. (1997) 'Health care in the United States', *Public Health Reports*, 112: 108–13.

Pollock, A.M., Macfarlane, A., Kirkwood, G., Majeed, F.A., Greener, I., Morelli, C., Boyle, S., Mellett, H., Godden, S., Price, D. and Brhlikova, P. (2011) 'No evidence that patient choice in the NHS saves lives', *Lancet*, DOI: 10.1016/S0140–6736(11): 61553–55.

Rechel, B., Wright, S., Edwards, N., Dowdeswell, B. and McKee, M. (2009) *Investing in Hospitals of the Future*, Copenhagen: World Health Organization.

Reich, M. and Takemi, K. (2009) 'G8 and strengthening of health systems: follow-up to the Toyako summit', *Lancet*, DOI: 10.1016/S0140–6736(08)61899–1.

Reich, M., Takemi, K., Roberts, M. and Hsiao, W. (2008) 'Global action on health systems: a proposal for the Toyako G8 Summit', *Lancet* 371: 865–69.

Shen, Y.-C. and Melnick, G. (2004) 'The effects of HMO ownership on hospital costs and revenues: is there a difference between for-profit and non-profit plans?' *Inquiry*, 41(3): 255–67.

Talbot-Smith, A., Pollock, A.M. and Gnani, S. (2004) 'Questioning the claims from Kaiser', *British Journal of General Practice*, 54: 415–21.

Timmins, N. (2001) *The Five Giants: A Biography of the Welfare State*, New York: HarperCollins, New Edition.

Van de Ven, W.P. (2011) 'Risk adjustment and risk equalization: what needs to be done?' *Health Economics, Policy and Law*, 6: 147–56.

Van de Ven, W.P., Beck, K., Buchner, F., Chernichovsky, D., Gardiol, L. and Holly, A. (2003) 'Risk adjustment and risk selection on the sickness fund insurance market in five European countries', *Health Policy*, 65: 75–98.

Walsh, K. (1995) *Public Services and Market Mechanisms: Competition, Contracting and the New Public Management*, Basingstoke: Macmillan.

WHO (2000) *World Health Report 2000*, Geneva: World Health Organization.

——(2006) *World Health Report 2006*, Geneva: World Health Organization.

——(2008) *World Health Report 2008*, Geneva: World Health Organization.

3 Rethinking problems surrounding access to care: the moral economies shaping health care workforces in Russia and the USA

Michele Rivkin-Fish

'With paid services, you get the best doctors,' explained the chief doctor of a Russian gynecology clinic, in reply to a question about the differences between paid and free abortions.

'Can you guarantee they're the best?'

'Well,' Valentina Pavlovna admitted, 'the women think there's a guarantee.' She paused, evidently uncomfortable with the ethical challenge the discussion raised. 'I can't do bad work,' she concluded with a tone of insistence. 'Sometimes I even do more for free than for those who pay.'

(Excerpt from fieldwork, St Petersburg, Russia, 1994)

'I would say that in general, there's that mentality, "you get what you pay for ... ." You know, I'm not saying I'm like that, or anybody else in here is ... but that's kinda ingrained in people when they purchase anything – services, or cars – you don't pay a lot, or nothing, you don't expect a lot ... '

(US dental student, in a large group conversation about the potential for compromises of care to occur in volunteer clinics for the poor, 2010)

The first conversation excerpted above took place in an era when for-fee provisioning of health care services was first being established as a central feature of Russia's broader, post-Soviet health care reforms. The second statement took place over a decade and a half later in the United States, just months after the Congress passed and President Obama signed historic legislation mandating comprehensive health care reform aimed at increasing coverage and affordability. Despite their separation in time and space, these excerpts reveal a common cultural contradiction that plays out in contexts of market-oriented health care. These two health professionals simultaneously confirmed and rejected an approach to the exchange of health care as analogous to the exchange of any other consumer service, an approach captured in the aphorism 'you get what you pay for.'

When the Russian clinic chief backtracked to assert, 'I can't do bad work,' she implicitly contested the widespread assumptions in health policy circles that physicians' 'interest' in the outcomes of their work is derived solely from how well they are paid.[1] For Valentina Pavlovna and many Russian doctors, at stake in the issue of whether women who paid actually obtained a superior quality of care was nothing less than their sense of professional pride and dedication. She had spent her entire career in the Soviet socialist model of free and universal health care, which charged physicians with the obligation of providing competent care to all patients for free as a matter of professional integrity. Yet she was reincarnating her clinic based on the popular notion that physicians' expertise and dedication was *only* available if *bought*.[2] Still, when asked directly about whether she endorsed inequalities of care based on ability to pay, she found herself unable to condone this practice as ethically acceptable.

The US dental student's statement is telling in that he phrased his perspective through caveats – 'I'm not saying I'm like that, or anybody else in here is ... but [the get-what-you-pay-for mentality is] kinda ingrained in people when they purchase anything.' Implicitly, he denied that, as a health care professional, he would provide compromised care to the poor – an admission that would seem to violate professional integrity if not also formal ethics. Yet at the same time, he suggested it would be reasonable for health care users to expect to receive worse quality care if they obtained those services for free or through reduced fees.

Health policy planners and analysts would do well to contemplate this ambivalence characterizing the relationship between users' fees, professionals' integrity, and the presumed unequal quality of medical care. This ambivalence, I will show, stems from mixed cultural messages and uncertain criteria about entitlement, or about what different groups of physicians and patients are seen to deserve. Tacit understandings about entitlement are linked with actors' expectations of their own and others' obligation and responsibility; these understandings in turn shape the kinds of claims perceived as legitimate, and the resulting silences that characterize certain kinds of need; they also work as logics shaping the ways providers conceptualize their career choices and daily work practice. Indeed, cultural visions regarding various groups' legitimate scope of entitlements and their related responsibilities stand in relation to each other in a systematic way and shape daily practice. Anthropologists refer to this interrelated set of concepts and practices as moral economies, or 'consensual assumptions about reciprocal obligations' (Minkler and Cole 1997: 40), understanding 'economies' here to involve the circulation of goods, both material (such as money and benefits) and non-material (such as dignity, integrity, entitlement, and social standing) – and noting how these various types of goods are often intertwined. We analyze the ways in which moral economies serve as the implicit conceptual backdrop against which certain cultural practices are reproduced without question as 'the right thing to do,' while other practices may be protested against as representing betrayals of justice or the violation of fairness (Thompson 1971).

My goal in this chapter is to introduce the framework of moral economies to the study of health care policy planning and analysis in Russia and the United States. More specifically, I suggest that efforts to improve access to care by addressing physician workforce issues have not adequately conceptualized the ways health providers' experiences, aspirations, and strategies are embedded in moral economies that define (if ambivalently and with contradictions) professional and patient entitlement and obligation. Examining the moral economies of health care and professional work through which providers in Russia and the United States make sense of their career decisions and daily practice will bring new and important insights into the challenges of increasing access to underserved populations.

Both Russia and the United States have great needs to extend access and improve the quality of health care. The particular characteristics of these two countries' health care systems and system needs are dramatically different: whereas Russia's problems of access stem from gaps in what is supposedly a universal model of free health care, the USA's system of work-based insurance structurally ensures that tens of millions of citizens will face barriers to access because of lack of health care coverage.[3] Russian health care reforms have focused on introducing new financing mechanisms while facilitating the emergence of private and semi-privatized services; in the USA, contrastingly, new health care reforms aim to extend insurance coverage and enhance the capacity of community-based, publicly funded clinics for rural and urban residents excluded by the market-based, private health care system.

While these differences are immensely important, it is also notable that, in both contexts, workforce issues entail a key part of efforts to address existing needs. In particular, health planners in both countries recognize that access and quality of care are intensely affected by the situations and actions of physicians. Yet in neither context do planners recognize how physicians' entanglement in access and quality of care issues is related to the moral economy of health care. This essay highlights the ways Russian and US physicians' career decisions and daily practices regarding patient access to their services are affected by culturally shaped notions of professional entitlement and patient worth, as well as the perceived symbolic worthiness of particular sectors of health care *vis-à-vis* the system as a whole. All of these are dimensions of the moral economy of health care.

The section that follows examines the ways Russian health policy planners and analysts have defined (and ignored) problems of access as they set about reforming their contemporary health care system. Mainstream discourses emphasize that barriers to access stem from doctors' demands for illegal payments from patients; and reforms focus on raising physicians' salaries. I then draw on my fieldwork, and more recent doctors' blog-postings, to argue that low salaries alone do not explain physicians' willingness to demand payments from patients – physicians draw on cultural and symbolic understandings of how medical work is and should be valued; they make social assessments of what kinds of persons they are treating, what kinds of care these patients deserve, and what these patients should offer in return for medical treatment. Such culturally embedded calculations, which often remain tacit or discussed through providers' jokes, stories, and the like, play a significant role in shaping the tenor and character of professional work. In other words, improvements in access and quality do not result mechan-istically from increased funding and higher salaries – because material issues alone do not capture the notions of entitlement and responsibility through which physicians make sense of their daily work practices. We need to see material remuneration as part of the broader symbolic messages that the state and patients communicate regarding the value of medical work and different forms of expertise; in turn, the actions of physicians can be seen as commentaries on the varying social worth of different patient groups, the perceived legitimacy of certain kinds of diseases, and their sense of what experts owe to patients, the state, and themselves.

I then turn to the US context, where health care reforms aim to promote physicians' and dentists' willingness to work in primary care and with under-served populations. Obama's reforms increase the funding for, and work opportunities in, primary care as a way of recruiting new graduates, while medical and dental schools undertake programs to cultivate students' com-mitments to 'communities' and 'service'. Yet public health clinics not only pay less, they also represent lower symbolic value relative to private practice. Market-based health care orients itself to the interests of consumers – those who pay for care – whereas recipients of public welfare services are deemed 'failed consumers', expected to be grateful for charity and not entitled to make demands. My fieldwork with dental students reveals how the disparate social worth of private and public clinics, their populations, and the mean-ings of work in each sphere get conveyed to new practitioners in training. Although committed faculty struggle to insist that under-served populations deserve high quality care, the structural organization of health care often confounds this message. Increased funding and pedagogical attention to the plight of the underserved importantly acknowledge the country's gaping inequities, but these reform efforts do not substantially subvert the moral economy of market-based medicine; such radical change would require the cultural acceptance of dramatically new calculations of clinician entitlement and the social worth of public health – a vision of clinicians as indebted to society for their training and opportunities, and a notion that all patients, regardless of social background, are entitled to high-quality services and dignity.

Understanding access to care and health care quality amidst Russia's reforms

The issue of health care access – ensuring that all patients who need medical care can receive it – is complexly intertwined with the transitions from a Soviet health care model to a post-Soviet one, whose financing procedures and legal guarantees are still being worked out some two decades after the collapse of the socialist system. Health care reforms are currently an official state priority, one of the 2006 National Projects that Putin established to reform governance and bring legitimacy to the state in the wake of several decades of massive cynicism towards decaying government services. The

1990s had witnessed an unprecedented public health crisis, characterized by skyrocketing rates of premature male mortality, plummeting fertility, the alarming spread of infectious disease, from tuberculosis to HIV, and more. While these indicators reflected the simultaneous confluence of multiple socio-economic disruptions and rapid cultural transformations, the Russian government also attributes part of the health care crisis to the poor funding and poor performance of the health care system itself (Ministerstvo 2009).[4] Citing the ongoing declining population numbers and extraordinary high rates of mortality, throughout the 1990s conservative and nationalist critics of market reforms accused the Yeltsin government of causing the 'genocide' of the Russian people, which, they claimed, was 'dying out' due in part to widespread unemployment, poverty, and a loss of social stability and values. Following this era, Putin built widespread legitimacy for his administration, in part through funneling portions of state revenues from higher oil prices into tangible benefits for citizens, especially through the partial revival of the state's withered system of social support. In the National Project for health care, these investments included increased funding to improve primary care, raise health care providers' salaries, build new medical clinics, and develop innovative methods and technologies – all represented as significant initiatives to improve the quality and accessibility of medical care (Antonova 2007: 191).

Given the fact that the Soviet health care system had one of the highest ratios of doctors to population in the world and a system of universal coverage, it is somewhat ironic that the country has been and continues to be plagued by serious problems of access at present. My ethnographic research and analysis of health policy debates in the 1990s found that barriers to access were created not only by financial need, but by pervasive cultural dynamics too: providers evaluated patients' social worth by assessing their apparent education and 'cultural level', as well as the type of condition patients had. Even at present, patients with HIV and other STIs face shaming and prefer to seek care at specialized AIDS centers rather than mainstream clinics (Bendina 2009). Exclusionary tactics against those deemed to have a 'low level of culture' are common, with the result that patients who felt berated distrusted the medical professionals and were reluctant to use their services (Rivkin-Fish 2005). Rusinova and Brown (2003) found that access to care depended on the networks and social skills that patients were able to deploy to maneuver around bureaucratic obstacles and pervasive mistrust. Patients' strategies, and their success in obtaining high quality services, differed according to their social strata and the related social and cultural capital they could mobilize. My research further explored the specific ways in which patients' strategies and networking affected providers' sense of personal obligations to provide especially attentive care. Close acquaintance relations facilitated access not merely to medical services, but even more importantly, to trustworthy, satisfying relations with providers. The acquaintance relationship in turn helped physicians, as they were more likely to have their expertise acknowledged and valued when they shared a personal connection with patients (Rivkin-Fish 2005). Certainly, personalized relations compromised the possibility of equity in health care; yet the perceived ethical character of these relationships, and the kinds of (inadequate) solutions they achieved to the problems of mutual distrust and enmity between doctors and patients, have not been addressed in policy debates, which often caricature these relations as simply exploitative and extortionist.

Until the late 1990s, many Russian health providers expressed great ambivalence about the introduction of fee-based health care, seeing required monetary payments as unethical and creating compromises in professional integrity. Physicians trained during the Soviet era described entering medicine as a calling, an arena in which scientific knowledge could be applied in an apolitical career that provided humanitarian-oriented workers with the satisfaction of saving lives. The financial remuneration was less than in other professional fields, but the sense of mission was invaluable. Yet, as Russian society underwent broader shifts driven by the profoundly transformative ubiquity of consumer culture, professionals began to redefine cultural expressions of self-respect, and their expectations for a dignified middle-class lifestyle transformed: markers of success (or failure) now became read in the clothing one wears, the mode of transportation one takes, the holiday destinations one chooses, the state of disrepair or remodeling of one's apartment. The significance of one's professional occupation became increasingly interpreted on the basis of whether it enabled culturally emerging aspirations to consume expensive goods. Male physicians told me their marriages were threatened because they were committed to practicing medicine in public hospitals and not demanding money from the poor; women physicians described being able to continue with their career only because they had 'rich' husbands who agreed to support their 'uncompensated' calling. Many worried about how they would fund their children's higher education as tuition payments were becoming more common. The economic crisis that medical professionals confronted was thus experienced as at the same time a piercingly unjust material deprivation, a traumatic source of life-altering interpersonal loss, and a cruel attack on the social value of their professional role.

The focus of health care reforms as early as 1993 centered on creating new financing models that would decentralize and shift the flow of resources away from the state as a monolithic funder. Policy makers roundly celebrated ideas of competition, fee-for-service, and salary differentiation for performance as solutions to the problems created by the Soviet system, almost never considering how market mechanisms in health care would affect access to care for the poor and socially marginalized or providers' own well-being. A brief examination of the actual realities wrought by this new financing model reveals both the ideological character of these reforms, and their narrow, mechanistic understanding of the social dynamics that shape access to care.

In the new financing system, employers and municipal governments were required to make contributions to quasi-governmental health insurance funds (OMC). Each of Russia's eighty-nine regions (except Chechnya) has its own fund, a situation that contributed to decentralized policies and significant variation across the country. The employer payroll tax for medical insurance of workers was set at 3.6 percent, an amount that both insurance fund directors and chief doctors decried as severely low, as reported in Judyth Twigg's survey conducted in 2000 (2002: 2260). Municipal governments made contributions on behalf of the non-working population. They determined their payments on a per capita basis, with the amount decided by each individual region (Twigg 2001: 204). The federal government was also to continue payments to health care, but the amount was small and expected to gradually diminish as an overall percentage of health care financing (Curtis et al. 1995: 760). In the year following Russia's financial crisis of 1998, the funding for health care as a proportion of GDP dropped by 30 percent (from 3.7 percent in 1997 to 2.6 percent in 1999); by 2007, it had risen to 3.5 percent of GDP (Ministerstvo 2009: 3). While the average per capita payment paid by regions was 5150 rubles, the actual amounts varied tremendously throughout the Russian Federation, from a low of 1723 rubles per capita paid in the Republic of Ingushetia to a high of 26,918 rubles per capita in Chukotka autonomous district (Ministerstvo 2009: 10).

In the early 2000s, Twigg noted that, in many regions, the OMC funds were working together with private insurance companies 'whose function is to guarantee the rights of patients and quality control' (Twigg 2002: 2254). Even at that time, head doctors and other critics questioned the usefulness of having insurance funds and private insurance companies, which represent an additional layer of administrative costs; concerns have been expressed that these companies were illegally diverting payments intended for the health care system for personal enrichment (Shchetinina 1999, quoted in Twigg 2002: 2261). In 2001, Twigg proposed somewhat vaguely that insurance companies seemed to be facilitating the collection of insurance taxes (2001: 217), but the mechanisms remained unexplained, and concerns continued that employers were not paying the full amount they owed. Indeed, referring to St Petersburg's reforms as early as 1995, Curtis et al. argued that:

> The involvement of private insurance companies will introduce an element of free market functioning and purchaser competition into the health insurance system. This is expected to be beneficial to the system, although the reasoning here may be more ideological than rational, since it is not altogether clear why the intermediary role of these agencies is necessary. It is difficult to see why the state public health administration, which has hitherto allocated budgets to health care providers, could not continue to use its expertise to spend the Fund for Health Insurance to purchase services directly.
>
> (Curtis et al. 1995: 760)

They suggested that the goal of creating these companies may have been to encourage a larger, independent health insurance market for individuals eventually to assume responsibility for their own health care (1995: 761).

Soviet and early post-Soviet Russian methods of financing of health care had occurred retrospectively, with state or insurance companies reimbursing clinics and hospitals for medical services delivered. With deficits in funds, debts accrued, and in the 1990s health care workers' already low salaries were delayed and demands for payments from patients increased (Twigg 2001: 205). The new health care financing scheme set budgets prospectively, allotting specific amounts of resources at the beginning of the budget cycle for a designated time period. 'Under these more planned circumstances,' Twigg suggested, 'the health care rationing presumably can take place according to medical need, rather than financial wherewithal' (2001: 205). Yet by 2007, it was clear that this form of rationing free medical care led federal budget makers and the OMC funds to establish strict quotas for the number of procedures for which they would pay, which actual patient needs far surpassed. As a consequence, patients faced the need to pay or refuse care (Antonova 2007: 192).

The fact that policy makers focused health care reforms on decentralizing financing and establishing markets, without assuming responsibility for the state to pay providers a respectable wage, led to important cultural shifts at the micro-level of everyday health care work. Providers' sense of what was ethically acceptable for them to do was rapidly shifting. After the financial crisis of 1998, physicians I knew who had earlier refused the idea of paid services now accepted them as necessary – and not for material reasons alone. They came to see monetary payment as an important symbolic acknowledgement that patients valued their expertise. The state had abandoned them, but individual patients still needed their services, and, many providers now told me, 'people find money for the things they value' (Rivkin-Fish 2009).

At the same time, providers suffered from a growing popular assumption among laypeople that physicians who remained in the public health care sector were those with poor skills, rather than fewer connections or interest in transferring to the private sphere. If Valentina Pavlovna, the clinic director described in the opening of this paper, exploited patients' assumptions that paying for services ensured access to the 'best doctors', physicians often felt stigmatized and less socially valued as a result of this worldview. Some described the array of medical cases at a public clinic as more interesting; others feared that patients at private clinics would be too demanding. Still others lacked the requisite contacts to seek work in semi-private clinics, or felt morally committed to public health care. In many of these cases, notions of what is at stake in one's work life – the interesting nature of the cases, the desirable characteristics of patients, or the ethical character of the health care provision – informed providers' career trajectories and daily work–life decisions. Physicians' calculations regarding what they sought out as valuable, and what they were willing to accept in return, were based on a complex combination of both material and social expectations – a moral economy.

Planners who expected physicians to work mechanistically for financial remuneration alone, and patients who assumed physicians toiling in public clinics were necessarily the least competent, failed to appreciate these complex desires, values, and aspirations.

In 2009, the Ministry of Public Health and Social Development of the Russian Federation issued a formal document of health planning, known as the Concept for the Development of the Public Health System for the Russian Federation through 2020.[5] This report revealed that the reforms to date had failed, in numerous ways, to promote higher quality or economic efficiency. The plan to have the OMC funds take over the bulk of health care financing did not come to pass, as in 2007 the federal, republic, and local municipal budgets were paying 63.4 percent of health care costs, while the OMC funds were providing 36.6 percent. The mere existence of OMCs, created as a signifier of decentralization, and the establishment of market mechanisms in health care, did not result in increased funding; rather, funding for the system languished until the federal budget increased its share of payments for health care following the creation of the 2006 National Projects. The inadequate funding resulted in several negative consequences for access to care and equity across social strata. While optional forms of fee-for-service care were being developed in select arenas of health care (such as abortion services, as noted above, dentistry, and maternity care; Rivkin-Fish 2005), the highly inadequate funding of the obligatory medical insurance funds resulted in a situation where unofficial users' fees were demanded for services that were supposed to be provided for free (Antonova 2007; Shishkin et al. 2007; Ministerstvo 2009). Nor did the new, decentralized payment entities improve the quality of care: 'The resources of the system of OMC are transferred to clinical treatment institutions through private insurance organizations (CMO), which are in no way interested in raising the quality of medical assistance for the insured or reducing expenditures for its provision' (Ministerstvo 2009: 10).[6]

Quantitative analyses of health care utilization, access, and coverage over the 2000s reveal enormous gaps and inequalities. Shishkin et al. (2007) found that the number of people who paid for outpatient medical services rose from 1994 to 2004 by 3.1 times, and for in-patient hospitalization by 3.4 times. After severity of illness, a patient's income was the most significant factor determining their seeking medical services: the rich (people in the fifth quintile of population) turn to doctors 37 percent more often than the poor (those in the first quintile) (2007: 16–17). The elderly were forced to wait longer for hospitalization, despite having two to three times the need for such care than working-age people (2007: 45). Nor was the new health insurance model universal: 10 percent of the population, mostly comprised of marginalized populations such as single men and unemployed, were not covered (Perlman et al. 2009). These researchers found that the widespread need to pay for medical care placed households from the poorest sectors of society at risk of 'catastrophic expenditures' in the case of severe illness;

people with chronic diseases faced barriers to accessing free services; and those in small towns were especially disadvantaged (Shishkin et al. 2007: 45). Often, patients were not informed about what they were officially entitled to receive: in a survey of patients in the city of Ekaterinburg, Antonova found that one-third of adult patients and a quarter of parents of children who were patients asserted that they were neither given the opportunity to get medical services for free, nor informed about the scope of their entitlements to seek it (Antonova 2007: 192).

Narratives explaining poor quality and inadequate access: mechanistic visions of provider behavior and the assumed magic of economic 'stimuli'

Despite these complex and multi-layered problems, the central narrative explaining barriers to access in Russia focuses on the low salaries of health care workers. Physicians' income levels are too low to cover their basic needs, as we will see in a selection from doctors' online postings below. The 2009 *Kontseptsiia* cites providers' low salaries as well as 'the equalizing approach to paying for medical personnel's labor, and the medical profession's low social protection and prestige … ' as causes for clinicians' 'weak motivation for professional perfection' (Ministerstvo 2009: 14). Indeed, providers' low salaries are consistently envisioned as motivating clinicians to demand illegal payments from patients (Antonova 2007; Shishkin et al. 2007). On November 24, 2009, the newspaper *Rossiiskaia gazeta* reported on the policy changes announced by the Concept paper. The article was picked up by the website start-capital.ru, which led with the headline, 'Salaries of doctors will rise in 2011', and opened with the following statement: 'From 2011 Russian doctors will begin receiving more money for their work with patients, and consequently will begin to treat patients better and extort less money for what are theoretically free services, the Federal Fund for Obligatory Medical Insurance promised … .' The Director of this Fund, Andrei Iurin, acknowledged that 'in the first half of 2009, the system of OMC received almost 26,000 complaints from citizens who were refused medical assistance and from whom monetary payments were unjustifiably demanded,' and promised that the new levels of funding would suffice to prevent these dynamics from continuing.

Moreover, both planners in the health financing system like Iurin, and scholars analyzing the dynamics of health care reform, call for economic stimuli to motivate physicians' clinical treatment of patients and use of health care resources. Iurin, for example, stated:

> … deep reforms are essential so that clinic doctors, hospitals and emergency vehicles do not refuse to treat patients who call upon them … For instance, a clinic doctor should receive a per capita fixed salary in relation to the population size, with additions adjusted to 'the real health' of the

population entrusted to him. The less frequently a patient needs to go to the hospital, call an ambulance, the better it will be for the patient and for the doctor ...

(Rossiiskaia gazeta 2009).

Shishkin et al. (2007) similarly advocate establishing per capita payments to 'interest' physicians in treating chronic diseases more effectively and efficiently (2007: 45). They advocate the creation of 'a list of the most widespread and socially significant illnesses to be treated according to federal and regional standards' (2007: 51). Yet they neither discuss the criteria for making such social and political judgments about which illnesses are socially 'significant,' nor recognize the inevitable exclusions that will ensue.

The mechanistic vision informing journalists and health policy analysts' recommendations is telling. The idea that financial stimuli will 'interest' health care providers in the outcomes of their work and automatically prevent the extortion of illegal payments (Antonova 2007: 196) relies on a model of provider behavior that ignores questions of how these professionals conceptualize responsibility, entitlement, and ethical action, and how various kinds of reforms may affect professionals' sense of participation in a moral economy of work. One set of health policy analysts refer to this cycle as based in providers' 'low morale' (Tkatchenko-Schmidt et al. 2010), a concept that speaks to the pervasive emotions health care providers express of frustration and abandonment. My point is that underlying these feelings is a logic of expert entitlement that has been experienced as violated; and so while raising salaries is important, it is necessary to understand the scope of entitlements and obligations perceived to be at stake. Do physicians believe that patients are always, or often, obligated to pay for their care because that which is free is not considered valuable? If so, what proportion of costs should they pay, and under what circumstances? To whom should they pay – the health care bureaucracy, the individual medical providers, or both? How do medical experts conceptualize their scope of responsibilities to patients, to the health care system, and to their profession? These questions are not addressed in health planners' reforms, and more research is needed to answer them. The following section examines how physicians' responses to the National Project convey their ambivalence towards both market mechanisms and the particular ways reforms have ensued in Russia. It offers a first step towards understanding physicians' notions of the moral economy of medical work.

Physicians' struggles between poverty and professionalism: seeking recognition of social worth

Physicians' cynical responses to the policy shifts announced in the 2009 *Kontseptsiia* conveyed their long-standing frustration with the state for failing to fund medical services. Certainly, their arguments advocate for salary increases, but they also reveal the multiple ways in which state wage levels are read as symbolic statements about social worth.

Among six postings on the website of Dmitrii Medvedev, President of Russia,[7] by physicians and others responding to the announced increase in salaries was a comment on May 2, 2010 from a male physician, who described himself as working in the state public health system since 1985 ...

> Respected Dmitrii Anatol'evich:
>
> ... a narrow specialist in an out-patient clinic gets a salary of 8–10,000 rubles a month, on average, while also providing consults in people's homes, answering these calls by walking there on his own two feet. Let's briefly count up the monthly expenditures for a family of 3 in which both parents are doctors: rent and utilities – 5000 rubles, phone – 500 rubles, transportation to and from work – 4000 rubles ... the child's transportation to school and lunch costs – 4000 rubles. Well, the sum already surpasses the salary, but there's still the need for money for the family's food, for clothes, for repairs to the school, for the child's text books. And more – you want to be a good doctor (indeed, you're answerable for a person's life), and in order to achieve that, you need to periodically go to unplanned courses to raise your qualifications, at the cost of between 20–50,000 rubles. What's more, internships in medicine cost 140,000 rubles a year!!! And a more or less decent medical textbook costs between 100–250,000 rubles! And you'd like to go on vacation at least once a year, to take your family to the beach, and that's another 100,000 rubles. Well, where is a simple doctor supposed to get this money? BECAUSE MEDICINE IN OUR COUNTRY IS FREE! Why then do you have to pay for bread, meat, and clothing? WELL, AND HOW ARE WE SUPPOSED TO LIVE? The fact is that the leaders of the country push doctors into the shadow economy of paid medical services. So you shouldn't chide us on this account. WE WANT TO WORK WELL AND RECEIVE A DIGNIFIED, OFFICIAL SALARY FOR THIS WORK!!! REAL IMPROVEMENTS IN THE CONDITIONS OF MEDICAL WORK, AND NOT JUST LIP SERVICE, ARE VERY DESIRED!!!

This posting captures the multi-faceted needs and aspirations of physicians: there are basic everyday material needs for the family as well as the need for a yearly vacation; and there is the need to be a competent professional capable of fulfilling the immense responsibility inherent in medicine – which requires funding for continuing education. The impossibility of achieving these needs on the basis of the state's official wages justifies providers' involvement in underground fee-for-service care, this author asserts. The language of his claim for a 'dignified, official salary,' and the framing of this claim as part of a set of reciprocal obligations in which physicians are to be held responsible as professionals for providing high-quality medicine, reveals aspects of the moral economy underlying providers' sense of their entitlements from the state, their obligations to patients, and their daily work decisions and strategies.

In another post on this site, a layperson named 'Olga1964' posted a commentary on December, 29, 2010 that captures the symbolism of comparative social worth at stake in evaluations of doctors' salaries:

> I don't understand why the governmental sector of the economy is being destroyed in our country ... How is it possible that doctors and teachers are paid 4–6000 rubles a month? Really, it's a mockery to pay kopeks for such difficult labor ... THEY at least understand what 5000 rubles means, when half of it has to be spent on the costs of rent and utilities, and the rest is what you have to live on for 30 days. And if a woman is a single mother? It would be interesting to know how much is spent for the jails to support prisoners. It would be interesting to know how many thousand rubles a little average parliamentary representative spends in a day. It would be interesting to lock up the parliament and feed them on 2000 rubles a month – would they survive for long? It would be interesting to raise the salaries by 10 percent (since to raise them by 6.5 percent is practically nothing): could they then be proud of themselves? Or should it be considered shameful? It would be interesting to know how much would be needed to increase doctors' and teachers' salaries by at least 100 percent. What percentage of the budget is allocated for rearmaments and Skolkovo?[8]

Another ninety-one people posted responses to the report on the website Start Capital, Guide to the Labor Market.[9] The selections below speak to the unease many providers continue to feel about the ethics of paid medicine, and their resentment of having to make the torturous decision of taking money from patients, working 'for free,' or leaving medicine. Lev, writing on February 18, 2011, stated:

> I am a generalist and a cardiologist ... The eternal question – Why did I go into medicine? Why am I still in medicine? If you work honestly, it's a terrible conveyor belt for mere kopeks, if you're sleezy, you feel bad about yourself. In commercial medicine they welcome sleeziness, if you work in the voluntary insurance sector – it's analogous to the state medical conveyor while keeping your eye constantly on the insurance company, and a CONSTANT ceiling for salary, even if you smash yourself to pieces. Plus fines.

Torn between his sense of ethics and the awareness that no sector of the health care system allows physicians to work according to their conscience and materially survive, Lev questions why he continues to stay in medicine at all.

Vladimir posted a comment on December 20, 2010 in which he described quitting medicine altogether in order to obtain a decent salary:

> I have 28 years experience as a doctor, I worked as an ophthalmologist in an outpatient clinic, first category. The salary was miserable. The chief doctor established an enormous daily production norm – 37 patients per shift ... In 2008 I stopped practicing medicine and now work as a house manager for a block of flats. The salary is three–four times more and I don't feel sorry about it at all. How can a specialist in pipes and garbage get paid a dignified salary, but doctors a minimum?

Those who remained also emphasized the ubiquitous compromises and perverse incentives that they confront in the market-based model of health care. Olga, for instance, posted on December 24, 2010:

> I have worked as a surgeon in an outpatient clinic for 25 years, highest qualification category. My salary rate is 6500 rubles per month, the rest are stimulus payments, which entirely depend on the good will of the administration. Every month a commission meets and determines the amount of the supplement. The decisive evidence of a doctor's work in our clinic is the fulfillment of the plan of for-fee services. Each doctor is given a plan for paid services, with each 1000 rubles in paid services, I get 130 rubles added to my salary. What do you think, are doctors interested in treating patients for free? Moreover, the insurance companies pay only for doctor visits in the clinics. That means that whether I operated or gave the patient a referral for analysis – the payment is the same. You want your furuncle operated on for free? Get it done at the hospital. Surgeons have become milking machines. And the scope of a doctor's responsibility? It is nonsense – a norm of six patients per hour, 36 per shift, 10 minutes per patient. They provide us with neither time, nor payment for surgical activities in the clinic. A question: does the outpatient clinic need surgical services? Or are we needed to insure the poor VOPa?

Similarly, another ophthalmologist, Liudmila, explained that financial benefits associated with 'paid medicine' are in practice linked to the good will of the clinic's administration:

> We have an enormous pool of patients – 850 persons per month, for whom we are paid kopeks. The salary scale is 4156 rubles, plus 30 percent of this scale for my tenure/experience, and five rubles for each patient above the norm. If you're reproached, you'll earn nothing. The stimulus payments which they promised 'will improve our lives' are 70 rubles per month for one point, and I have 12, so it totals 840 rubles, if 'I don't wrong anyone'.

Summary: physician workforce trends, health care access and quality – looking beyond low salaries to the moral economy of medical work

Doctors' seething anger at their miserly salaries defines their wages as unfairly low in relation to the basic costs of living, their rightful entitlement to a 'dignified' lifestyle, as well as the expenses they bear for continuing education costs to improve their knowledge. They regard their salaries as unfairly low in comparison with the wages of other professions that require lower qualifications. They criticize their high workloads as measured by the expected number of patients they must treat per month, per hour, and per shift, and by the extensive paperwork they need to complete. Several criticize the financial bonuses established for serving paying patients as leaving them 'uninterested' in providing 'free' care to the majority; others mention that the bonuses were not founded in a system of clear and transparent criteria for quality, but were subject to caprice and favoritism. Some speak of leaving medicine and not looking back; others of persuading their children against going into medicine and regretting that they personally remained in it.

The need for higher salaries is clear: but health care planners often overlook that salaries are not only material resources, but also symbolically important ones. Salaries convey a degree of respect, a sense of importance and value that all of the clinicians who wrote commentaries felt bereft of. Arguments that conceptualize the need for higher wages alone don't answer the key questions at stake for physicians and society at large: what is a fair salary for medical professionals? How should it be determined? Should physicians who work with wealthy patients earn more than those who work with poor patients? Or should the reverse be true? Should there be a 'bonus' for physicians who work with infectious patients, as there has conventionally been in Russia's health care system? How should the need to convey the value of medical work for stigmatized populations be balanced with the risk of entrenching stigma that such patients are 'dangerous'? Should physicians be compensated for patients who are kept healthy? Should they be paid per procedure, an incentive structure that may prompt unnecessary treatment? How should society balance the need for medical care among a highly impoverished population with the need for highly educated and skilled professionals to receive sufficient compensation to feel 'dignified' in a context where conspicuous consumption is increasingly idealized? How to define compensation in the healing professions so that new professionals' interests in caring for people are not eclipsed by mercenary goals, and the conflicts of interest that arise when medicine becomes a business remain in check? Health planners and policy analysts in Russia may be aware of these dilemmas, but a sustained dialogue between them and their employees, as well as society, has yet to occur.

Health care reforms in the United States: understanding access to care through the moral economy of professional workforce trends

The prevailing notion that markets best achieve labor force needs has meant that the USA has no centralized governmental body charged with deliberative workforce planning. Yet in the 1960s and 1970s, the US government recognized that the uneven distribution of physicians and dentists throughout the country constituted an abiding source of health disparities and social inequality. Since that time, a number of federal and state programs, as well as initiatives by private foundations, have been established with the goal of affecting workforce trends and improving these dynamics. Incentive programs encourage health professional students to choose primary care; encourage graduating generalists to serve rural populations and poor residents of inner cities; promote medical and dental education among minorities and students from rural areas, who are seen as more likely than whites and urban residents to serve these populations voluntarily; encourage private practitioners to accept the state insurance system of Medicaid, which reimburses at rates far lower than those of private insurance; and encourage health professionals from all disciplines and specialties to volunteer to help the uninsured access health care. In one of the first such initiatives, President Nixon signed legislation known as the Emergency Health Personnel Act of 1970 (Public Law 91-623), which established the National Health Service Corps (NHSC). This agency has been sending allopathic and osteopathic physicians, dentists, nurse practitioners, physician assistants, and certified nurse midwives to practice in areas where the population suffers from inadequate access to health care since 1972. The program offers scholarships and loan-repayment programs as incentives for professionals to work in these remote or underserved urban regions. Recipients of NHSC support make a minimum two-year commitment to working in officially designated health professional shortage areas; the agency currently has over 8000 health care providers serving over 7 million people and, with health care reform, the need for clinicians in these centers is expected to double.[10] Focusing on dentistry specifically, The Robert Wood Johnson Foundation initiated a national program in 2001 entitled The Pipeline, Profession, and Practice: Community-Based Dental Education (Dental Pipeline), to help increase the availability of oral health services for underserved communities. The program focused on dental education and training experiences, aiming to promote students' interest and competencies in working with underserved communities, and to recruit future providers, including minority and low-income students, into dentistry.[11]

However, over thirty years since this program was established, many of the problems identified in the mid-twentieth century continue to plague American health care. Inadequate supplies of the primary care workforce, the geographic maldistribution of providers, and widespread reluctance by practitioners to accept the state's insurance program of Medicaid continue.

President Obama's Patient Protection and Affordable Care Act of 2010 recognizes that addressing these long-standing problems is key to reforming the country's health care system. This Act's goal of expanding insurance coverage and health care access to the vast majority of the country's uninsured (currently estimated to be 50 million people) requires a massive increase in primary care professionals to serve these patients. This legislation invests significant resources in the recruitment of primary care professionals, funding residencies in primary care medicine, dentistry, and allied health professions,[12] increasing Medicare and Medicaid reimbursements for preventive care and chronic disease treatment,[13] funding loan forgiveness programs for health providers who work in underserved areas,[14] and supporting the community health centers that employ these providers to serve many rural and distressed urban populations.

These initiatives are certainly welcomed by advocates for underserved communities and proponents of health care reform. They represent important opportunities for students and practitioners with an interest in providing primary care to underserved populations to learn about these career trajectories and to gain the financial resources, social networks, and pragmatic knowledge necessary to do so successfully. Yet, beyond assisting those who are already oriented towards primary care, it is arguable that financial incentives alone will not result in the significant kinds of cultural transformations necessary to shift health professional workforce trends towards a massive influx of primary care and commitment to underserved populations. Cultural practices and ideologies in medical school and graduate medical education shape the development of workforces by establishing the varying social worth of primary care or subspecialties. Scholars of health care workforce dynamics are well aware that specialty medicine enjoys not only greater remuneration, but also greater prestige than primary care; and despite curricular reforms in undergraduate medical education that include attention to the social and cultural dimensions of health care and healing, academia has been described as creating a 'chilly climate' for those students interested in pursuing careers in primary care (e.g. Block et al. 1996). This is ironic, given that faculty at medical schools tend to be supporters of primary care education and practice. Yet surveys of faculty have found that even they deride generalists as less competent than specialists to care for patients with serious illness; they characterize research in primary care as low quality, and encourage capable medical students to pursue advanced training in more prestigious specialty disciplines. And the structure of graduate medical education reflects this ideology of social worth: the administrations of teaching hospitals make decisions about the amount of positions to create in different fields, and trends have focused on reducing those in generalist fields such as family medicine while increasing positions in subspecialty residencies. The guiding concerns comprise not public health needs but institutions' own priorities (Goodman 2008: 1206), including prestige, projected revenue, etc.

Nor is this to say that the financial dimensions of career choice are unimportant: one study found that medical students accrue on average approximately $124,000 of debt, with a substantial number (18.5 percent) facing over $200,000 of debt. Dental students' debt was at similar levels.[15] Students consider the burden of debt they will face when making practice decisions, and the salary differentials between primary care and specialties are great: family medicine practitioners had the lowest average annual salary of all physicians, reaching $186,000 in 2007, while orthopedic surgeons averaged $436,000 that year (Ebell 2008). Health planners rightly argue that these disparities affect the exceedingly low proportion of US medical student graduates who choose primary care work (family medicine, pediatrics, and general internal medicine), the latter reaching a low of 2 percent of all graduates in 2007 (Hauer et al. 2008). Indeed, many students describe the immense financial debt they accrue as justifying the choice of lucrative specialties practices, to ensure their ability to repay loans while still achieving the high standard of living they feel entitled to enjoy.

My argument, as in the Russian case discussed above, is that remuneration is much more than materially significant – it must be seen as part of the logic of professional obligations and entitlements that I describe as the moral economy of medical work. Health professional training teaches students not only the technical competencies of their future careers, but also an understanding of the scope of obligations they have to their patients and society at large, and the entitlements they can legitimately expect in return, from pay and benefits to workload and lifestyle. In contrast to formal bioethics frameworks that articulate universal standards of professional ethics for all institutional contexts and patient populations, the uneven distribution of symbolic and material capital in the medical field actually results in divergent kinds of expectations, entitlements, and practices for different arenas and populations of practice. In other words, students learn to read (and often accept) the inequalities structured into society (and specifically our health care system) as signs of various social groups' and medical arenas' unequal social worth. Professional socialization, what might be called the creation of new providers' subjectivities, involves learning to see oneself as part of that health care system, a process that involves making personal calculations in relation to these dominant notions of disparate social worth. Students establish their goals, sense of obligations, entitlements, and career and life expectations in terms connected with the kinds of value they place on medicine's divergent fields of practice, institutional settings, specialties, and patient populations, as well as the kinds of obligations they may have in their personal life.[16] Inasmuch as work in primary care brings low symbolic capital relative to specialty work, and underserved populations are also often stigmatized groups, students recognize that providers who work in these arenas are precariously positioned in terms of dominant notions of social worth, status, prestige – as well as receiving lower pay. Health planners need to recognize that these broader dimensions of the moral economy of medical work are key stakes for professionals who consider primary care and work with the underserved.

My fieldwork analyzes the cultural project of defining and creating the ethical health professional in the US context of market health care, with its increasing inequities. While didactic instruction focuses on technical and clinical skills, students and residents continually acquire knowledge about potential ways in which they may interface with the health care system, including its public arenas and underserved populations. In the process, many form professional subjectivities that are suited to the moral economy of American market-based health care, with its notions of varying social worth among populations and practice sites. As I show in the case study below,[17] health professional programs that strive to generate students' professional commitment to the underserved often unintentionally reproduce dominant messages about the differential social worth of private and public institutions and recipients of care. These programs celebrate altruism and empathy, and highlight a vision of health care as a service as well as a 'business'. Yet community-based programs are also situated within the broader socialization process shaped by the US moral economy of health care, characterized by unequal opportunities for poor patients and the unquestioned societal respect for professional choice and entitlement in career and practice decisions. Professional obligations are narrowly defined in terms of ethical responsibilities to individual patients, and rarely oblige providers to address health care inequities. With this grounding set of assumptions, students are positioned as entitled to make personal choices without a sense of being indebted to society and obliged to make returns in their professional work.[18] This broadly based consciousness informs students' community-based encounters with the underserved, and is reconfirmed by their structured relationships with poor people in these programs. As a result, students may come away from their community-based learning experiences with their pre-existing stereotypes about the low value of public health clinics, and the distasteful character of underserved populations, reaffirmed.

The second quotation at the opening of this chapter exemplifies this perspective. In 2010, I led a large group conversation with eighty US dental students and faculty on the question of 'Why we volunteer', in which I asked participants to discuss their motivations and to address whether they saw volunteer work as resulting in compromised standards of care. In stating that the mentality, 'you get what you pay for ... ' is 'ingrained in people', this student reminded his peers and supervisors that patients who do not have private insurance or the personal funds to pay for services will receive lower-quality care, rendering this reality a fact of life, even if – in the same sentence – he implicitly acknowledged that this stance was ethically questionable for health care providers to embrace towards their patients – 'I'm not saying I'm like that, or anyone else here is ... '.

When dental students work in community-based clinics, they witness the routine provision of substandard care to patients who have no insurance coverage or the government sponsored health insurance, Medicaid.[19] Whereas at dental school students learn that the appropriate form of care involves undertaking all efforts to restore decayed teeth, they find that community clinics regularly extract potentially restorable teeth because Medicaid does not pay for fillings or root canals, only for extractions, and patients are unable or unwilling to pay for restorations themselves. This policy clearly creates treatment disparities based on patients' finances, and leads to negative implications for the oral health status of poor people as edentulism often results. But this policy also conveys the state's low regard for the adult poor as undeserving recipients of high-quality dental services. (Notably, Medicaid covers children's restorations and preventive care, revealing that children, unlike adults, are considered deserving of state support.) This policy, and the routine forms of treatment that result from it, position poor patients and the clinics that specialize in their care as symbolically inferior and less socially valuable than private practice patients and providers.

Thus, alongside explicit messages depicting community-based work as virtuous, students also learn how the broader dental profession and public policy makers assign value to various spheres of practice and the participants in them. By the time students undertake required rotations in public health clinics after their third year of studies, they are well aware of the structural and symbolic distinctions between public health and private practice dentistry. They are familiar with the pejorative concepts of the 'public health mentality,' and stereotyped 'Medicaid clinic' images that they described to me as conjuring up poorly equipped, poorly skilled, and cynical clinicians who supposedly work as little as they need to, or even engage in unscrupulous practices.[20] They are well versed in discourses that portray poor patients as unreliable, failing to show up for appointments, non-compliant, and apathetic about their oral health. They know that private practice, by contrast, is widely considered the norm of success, where a dentist chooses his or her clientele, earns well, and enjoys autonomy.

It is crucial to note, however, that many of the professionals who work with underserved populations have developed alternative narratives about both the value of their work for society, and the dignity, respect, and entitlements of their patient populations. When supervising students, they serve as role models for these alternative ways of understanding social worth, and partly redefine the moral economy of professional obligations. Moreover, students observe the ways their faculty members and clinic-based preceptors interpret and relate to this systematic form of inequality, learning possible ways to construe and manage their relationships with patients within this stratified system. These alternative discourses – along with increased salaries and improved work conditions – are the necessary symbolic shifts that need to occur for primary care and work with underserved populations to become more valued and to be taken up as career choices by new graduates.

Clinic staff who have devoted their lives to underserved communities negotiate the ideology of social worth as part and parcel of their daily work lives. They contest the portrait of their clinic as second-rate, and insist that their patients are entitled to the same respect and quality of care as any other patient. Dr Davis, an African-American woman who directed a not-for-profit pediatric clinic, told me:

> Because so many patients and parents who are on Medicaid have been made to feel like second class citizens … from day one, our philosophy was that we want them to feel the same way when they're coming into our office as if they were going into any private office in the area. We did not want them to come here and feel like, 'Oh this is a clinic for Medicaid patients, oh, this is a clinic for poor kids.' We didn't want that stereotype or that stigma. So from the very beginning our staff has gone over and beyond and rolled out the red carpet to make parents feel good when they come here.

In stating at the outset that Medicaid recipients 'have been made to feel like second class citizens', Dr Davis alluded to entire sets of social forces that have created barriers to patients' health. She took responsibility for the ways her institution interacted with patients, creating policies that drew on extensive knowledge about her patients' lives, and ensuring the students she supervised understood the difficulties they faced in trying to access dental services without a car or a flexible job. She taught students who interned at her clinic that she expected all staff to treat her patients with respect, and she modeled a collaborative form of interaction with parents to ensure that they could access the care their children needed. Yet, ironically, Dr Davis' description of her strategy invoked the image of the stereotypical 'Medicaid clinic' and accepted the symbolic dominance of 'private practice' clinics as the gold standard of social worth. She insisted that this model was the entitlement of her patients, just like those with private forms of payment.

The moral economy of professionals' entitlement and choice

Numerous conceptual barriers limit the extent to which alternative discourses can succeed in redefining primary care and work with the underserved as genuinely socially valuable. Among them, as we have seen, are the lower pay and reimbursement levels, the (debatable) assumption that primary care is technically unsophisticated, and the stigma that often attends poor populations. Another dimension of the moral economy of the US health care system that bears discussion is the pervasive sense of entitlement that health professional students learn to have regarding their own career trajectories and priorities. This stance is structured into health professional training. Some dental school faculty recognize this unmitigated entitlement as a problem, as Dr Stevens told me: 'The state gives funding for dental education. Students' education is partly paid for by tax dollars, so they should have an obligation to give back to the community. Yet they don't realize it, for they take out so much in loans they aren't thinking about how their education is subsidized.' Still, it is notable how little attention is paid to the idea that students should contribute to the public's health and welfare, given the investment of tax revenue in health professional education (for a rare exception to this trend, see Goodman 2008).

My interviews and fieldwork revealed that students almost always receive the opposite message – that they are free to choose how to practice dentistry and to prioritize whatever personal goals they have. One of the ways students received this message was seen in how volunteer work for the underserved was structured. Dental schools provide extensive support for these community programs through donations of equipment and materials, and by recognizing (if not often paying) faculty supervision of students in student-run clinics and mobile dental clinics. Working in such clinics comes after a long day of classes and on weekends; it often involves arduous work with patients whose lack of comprehensive care results in multiple medical complications. To work in mobile dental clinics, students often get up as early as 4:00 a.m. and drive for three hours to remote parts of their state, in order to be available for some of the hundreds of patients who have been waiting outdoors all night for an opportunity to obtain free services at the one-time clinic.

Dental students and others hoping to attend dental school in the future make significant contributions to these clinics. I attended two all-day clinics provided by an organization called Devoted Dentists and Supporters (DDS), along with members of a dental student volunteer organization, 'Students for Smiles.' One clinic was in an inner city area, the other in a small rural town, which opened its doors to patients from areas as far as a five-hour drive away. The dental faculty and student service organization recruited participants and nurtured a collective sense of camaraderie throughout these clinic events. A 'do-good' spirit of volunteerism characterized participants' mood, who described the work as 'fun' and 'rewarding.'

In interviews I conducted with students and faculty members, I learned about the moral economy underlying many students' interest in undertaking volunteer work with underserved populations. A faculty member who supervised these programs, Dr Natalie Osborne, discussed her strong concerns that many students volunteered for 'a chance to seek independence and not have the supervision they have at the dental school clinic. They want to try things out and see what they can do. But that's not what this is about.' It was an open secret that students participated in the mobile clinics with expectations of doing 'exciting' technical procedures, and Dr Osborne worried that these motivations were both ethically misguided and potentially dangerous, as students may not have the skills to carry out specific procedures, especially on patients with numerous complications in substandard clinic conditions – the mobile units had poor lighting and substandard equipment relative to the dental schools where students were training, and the atmosphere was bustling, with the pressure of hundreds of patients waiting on bleachers for a turn to receive treatment. In addition, Dr Osborne also confronted students' reluctance to do procedures that they considered less interesting, such as teeth cleaning. When I interviewed Dr Marshall, an active organizer of the DDS clinics, he described his strategy of making participation in the mobile clinics desirable for students:

> We make it fun for the kids so they want to come, not like school. I do my damnedest to make it no pressure. I let them do what they want to do – let them feel, experience themselves as practitioners. You know, we give them supervision and everything ... Some students go on repeat basis. It makes a difference. I know that some have decided to take Medicaid in their private practice or work in public health departments.

As I learned in the course of fieldwork, this statement was an allusion to the fact that the DDS organizers were encouraging and supervising students in doing extractions, even if they had not yet qualified academically to do so. The 'excitement' of getting to try one's hand at new procedures was the return students would receive for the sacrifice of their time to the volunteer clinic. This exchange did not go uncontested – Dr Osborne fought to establish strict limits on student participation and supervision – but the case exemplifies a broader structural relationship in which students come to experience their career as built on choices and opportunities, and may never question the substandard care and inequities structured into services for the poor. Dr Marshall, it must be noted, was far from indifferent about the interests of poor and underserved communities. He had dedicated his career as a dentist to serving the poor, and he realized that mobile clinics were at best a band-aid on a gaping wound of inadequate oral health care. But he was proud that they created a venue to treat thousands of poor patients, and brought the plight of the underserved to public attention. He also saw the clinics as an opportunity to create enthusiasm for public service among the upcoming generation of dentists, a generation whose choice of career trajectories generally did not seem to develop out of concerns for collective well-being.

This sense of professional entitlement was pervasive. At a closing ceremony for dental students in her state, Dr Davis addressed the newly graduating dentists by advocating for the underserved. Her comments, framed in the genre of a motivational talk, illustrate this aspect of the moral economy organizing health care workforce trends in the United States:

> You can have a successful practice and still provide dental health care to underserved populations. 'You can have it all.'
>
> ... Dentistry is a wonderful profession, and I consider it a privilege to have been called to do it. And I do believe it is a calling. Everyone can't do what we do. So it is incumbent upon us, by virtue of being able to have the opportunity to practice in such a great profession, to say thank you by 'giving back.'

Let me share a story with you about one underserved person. This is an excerpt from *The Washington Post* dated February 28, 2007:

'Twelve-year-old Deamonte Driver died of a toothache Sunday. The bacteria from the abscess had spread to his brain, doctors said. After two operations and more than six weeks of hospital care, the Prince George's County boy died. A routine, $80 tooth extraction might have saved him. If his mother had been insured. If his family had not lost its Medicaid. If Medicaid dentists weren't so hard to find' (Otto 2007).

Just how bad is this access to care issue for the poor and underserved?

The [state] Medical Journal reports that ... there are as many as forty counties where there is no dentist willing to serve a Medicaid patient. Dental Medicaid, as you know, is the dental insurance program designed by the state and federal government to pay for dental treatment for low-income individuals. Fewer than one in three Medicaid recipients sees a dentist each year.

Why don't more dentists sign up for Medicaid? One of the reasons that dentists don't sign up for Medicaid is because of the low reimbursement rates, which range from 35 percent to 85 percent of what the dentist charges based on the 2007 National Dental Advisory Service median.

An active Medicaid dentist (as defined by the Division of Medicaid Assistance) is one who receives at least $10,000 dollars in Medicaid reimbursements per year.

I can hear you saying: 'Dr Davis, this all sounds good and altruistic, and it's giving me warm fuzzies, but you must be going bonkers! How can I make my annual production goals if I see any Medicaid patients? How would I combat the no-show problem? I can't do it, I have too much debt.' And I know, I know, some of your mentors have warned you against taking Medicaid, but if the tide against providing access to care is to change, it must change with you!

According to the 2005 American Dental Association Survey of Dental Practice, the average US dental office has almost $600,000 in gross billings per year. Providing $10,000 in Medicaid care would come to less than 2 percent of gross charges per year.

You can have it all and still give back to your community!

This passage is interesting in the way it critically exposes the fatal injustice generated by the US dental system, challenges practitioners to take responsibility for changing that system, and still underscores practitioners' privileged position within the moral economy of market-based health care. Dr Davis opens her speech by asserting that it is 'incumbent upon us ... ' to say thank you by 'giving back'. She celebrates dentistry as a 'great profession', linking her audience's personal and professional pride with a general sense of obligation beyond themselves. She then recounts the depth of need and the consequences of gaps in care to poor populations through the story of a twelve-year-old boy who died due to an untreated tooth infection. The boy's death could have been averted 'If his family had not lost its Medicaid. If Medicaid dentists weren't so hard to find.' With this quote from *The Washington Post*, Dr Davis holds dentists accountable for this boy's preventable death, and she continues to explain that financially, a commitment to providing $10,000 a year in Medicaid services would have minor effects on an average practice's profitability.

Despite presenting this ethically troubling account of professional and policy complicity in the creation of dire inequalities, the tone and thrust of this talk is neither accusatory nor shaming, but celebratory and inspirational. It emphasizes dentists' entitlement and privilege, and explains that a modest commitment to working with the underserved will bring substantial emotional returns to the dentists themselves. Dr Davis' theme, the refrain she returns to again and again in this talk, is that dentists 'can have it all' – financial success and the rewarding feeling of 'giving back'. The sacrifice is modest; the reward, substantial.

As a mode of encouraging private practice dentists to dedicate a minimal amount of their regular workload to patients with Medicaid, this rhetorical strategy exposes how thoroughly naturalized the moral economy of American dentistry is: just as the entitlement of 'having it all' rhetorically supersedes the obligation to 'give back' in terms of its emphasis in the speech, we can also trace how the solution to the dire problems of health care access relies on maintaining dentists' entitlement to satisfaction. Certainly, this rhetoric makes strategic sense given the broader political–economic context in which it is embedded, where members of the dental profession historically have opposed state efforts to limit their professional autonomy, opposed state programs for insurance coverage, opposed norms of 'universal patient acceptance',[21] remained largely unmoved by the low reimbursement rates of Medicaid, and at present increasingly work in specialties of aesthetic and cosmetic dentistry, despite the massive numbers of Americans without access to primary dental services. Advocates for social justice in health care deploy multiple strategies for change, at times pushing against the moral economy that allocates lower social worth to the poor, but often working within that system, highlighting, for example, the feel-good rewards that come with providing community service. Their battles need to be recognized and supported.

Conclusion

I opened this chapter by highlighting the ambivalence providers express about the ethics of providing differential standards of care based on patients' ability to pay – an ambivalence that coexists with claims for better pay in Russia and a sense among US health professional students that their burden of student debt entitles them to seek the most lucrative specialties. My point has been that efforts to motivate health care providers to serve the poor, and those with unaddressed primary care needs, must conceptualize money as part of a symbolic package of value, not merely a material good. The reshaping of workforce trends would require nothing less than the transformation of dominant assumptions of social worth and deservingness, so that poor patient populations, public venues for care, and primary care forms of expertise become treated as highly valuable contributions to society.

For all its inadequacies, the Soviet health care system had cadres of professionals who saw themselves as obliged to serve; the acceptance of monetary payment for medical care was a sign of physicians' personal and bureaucratic corruption, greed, and failure to realize socialist welfare principles. This stance has eroded over the past two decades, eclipsed by notions that payment is a sign of well respected work and that people will find money for things that they value (regardless of their financial situation) (Rivkin-Fish 2009). Contemporary Russian health planners aim to improve the quality of health care in part by instituting monetary incentives for providers' 'quality work'. Economic stimuli for professionals are widely accepted as a necessary corrective to Soviet-era egalitarian approaches to remuneration, which are considered to have provided a disincentive for hard work and continual personal improvements.[22] Yet the system of incentives undermines the cultural ideal that patients are entitled to free services; and it leaves providers with no clear path for ethical practice, for there is no longer a clear understanding of what constitutes professional integrity in terms of payment for services, no clear way to be fair to one's patients and oneself. Moreover, existing methods of determining employees' worthiness to receive extra pay are perceived to be unfair and mired in favoritism, displays of deference, and quality-compromising patient volume quotas.

US health care reforms also aim to change workforce trends by making substantial financial investments in primary care, seeking to motivate new practitioners to work in these fields and with underserved populations. Certainly, this funding is important. Yet deliberative dialogues and public debate regarding what kinds of medical work are valued and why; what responsibilities physicians have to their patients, their clinical institutions, their society; and what they are owed – by patients, their institutions, and society – remain severely unexamined. As tens of millions of US citizens may obtain access to health insurance in the coming years, health care workforce development continues to be based on voluntary choice and institutional, not public health-focused, priorities. Recruitment efforts for staffing clinics in health professional shortage areas will likely become urgent. The cultural discourses and rhetoric infusing these efforts not only will shape their immediate success in attracting professionals, but will impact the kinds of expectations, obligations, and entitlements that motivate those providers who choose to work with and for the poor.

In both neoliberal contexts, the notion that physicians should be paid on the basis of 'their performance' remains an ideological statement rooted in a mechanistic vision that money stimulates hard work and 'quality,' without extensive consideration of the conflicts of interest at stake, including: how to prevent the profit motive from generating overuse or underuse of medical treatment; and how to balance personal financial incentives with commitments to individual patients, while also developing a sense of institutional stewardship for collective resources. Nor does this vision address the sense of professional pride and integrity, and the multiple, often competing concerns that can arise when professional pride stems from technological competence and prowess, rather than humanitarian concerns to recognize patients as more than their disease, and from dedication to alleviate patient suffering.

Envisioning health care systems and workforce trends as rooted in 'moral economies' moves us away from discussions of provider 'attitudes' and 'choices' conceptualized as aggregates of individual sentiments, priorities, and values. The lens of moral economies highlights how 'attitudes' and 'choices' are embedded in broader social structures that position people to have certain kinds of interests, entitlements, and related understandings of their scope of obligation in the variety of roles they assume. It offers an analytic framework that captures how health care systems and public policies allocate differential social value to varying arenas of health care practice and populations seeking care; such unequal value may impact health professionals' calculations about their careers and their decisions about their daily practices. The concept of moral economies offers a new way to conceptualize the relationship between health professional workforce dynamics and access to care for the under-served, and it promises to open up dialogue about the kinds of obligations and entitlements that we want our professionals to have, that we want health care users to have, and the forms of social worth we will recognize.

Notes

1 This quote, notably, exposed the fact that the deregulation and creation of a consumer market in Russian health care has not led simply to a higher quality of care. Clinics exploited the widespread patient dissatisfaction with the quality of free care, combined with the lack of public information about health care reforms and the lack of state oversight, to turn a profit.

2 One could argue that it would be possible to discern levels of physician quality. Yet in mid-1990s Russia, there was no systematically collected measuring of data or comparing of physicians' 'quality' (or dedication). The notion of what constituted the 'best doctors' had not been subject to rational analysis or public discussion, but was being 'sold' as a desirable commodity.

3 Additionally, anti-immigration politics ensure that millions of non-citizens will be excluded from accessing health insurance (Galarneau 2011).

4 The state's own analysis asserts: 'Between 1991 and 1994, as a result of the substantial reduction in the population's standard of living, life expectancy decreased by five years. Following the financial crisis of 1998, which led to a 30 percent reduction in the expenditures on public health (from 3.7 percent of GDP in 1997 to 2.6 percent in 1999), the average life expectancy decreased by 1.84 years. The increase in life expectancy between 2005–7 was, to a significant degree, linked to the increase in expenditures on medical assistance, which rose from 2.6 percent of GDP in 2005, to 2.9 percent of GDP in 2007, and in expenditures on public

health overall, which rose from 3.2 percent of GDP in 2005 to 3.5 percent of GDP in 2007' (Ministerstvo 2009: 3).

5 www.zdravo2020.ru/concept

6 State planners and insurance experts at times acknowledge the conflicts of interest inherent in market-based health care, as the following two examples indicate. Yet in neither case do the authors follow up their concessions with calls for regulations or modifications to prevent such compromises from occurring. The Kontseptsiia acknowledges: 'An additional channel of resources for treatment-prevention institutions is paid medical services and the program of individuals' voluntary medical insurance (DMC). The presence of these sources, on the one hand, allows these clinics (in cases of insufficient financing) to receive additional resources for the salaries of its workers and the continual maintenance of the clinic, but, on the other hand (in the absence of rigid regulation of these services), leads to the reduction in access and quality of medical care for the population that are served in the program of government guarantees' (Ministerstvo 2009: 10). A specialist at a medical insurance company explained: 'Paid medicine is bad in that, in making medical services a business, it leads to hyperdiagnosis and overuse of services. A doctor who is interested in increasing the number of appointments and diagnostic procedures will prescribe, often in agreement with his partners, a greater amount of procedures that are not justified' (Antonova 2007: 194).

7 www.mailpresident.ru/node/5037

8 A planned high-tech business area in Moscow Oblast.

9 www.start-capital.ru/news/1930.html?p=1#comments

10 http://nhsc.hrsa.gov/about/history.htm; see Trude, *Laura Health Workforce News*, September 2010. http://hwic.org/news/sept10/curtin.php

11 http://dentalpipeline.org/elements/community-based/pe underserved.html

12 Patient Protection and Affordable Care Act of 2010 (PPACA), sections 5101–5601 (United States Congress 2010).

13 PPACA sections 2703 and 3502.

14 PPACA section 3013.

15 In 2001, a dental graduate's average amount of debt totaled $113,000 (Haden et al. 2003: 573).

16 Both media and scholarly accounts note that the increasing number of women entering the health professions has coincided with a growing interest among professionals to prioritize their 'lifestyle' concerns in career decisions, as compared with earlier generations of physicians whose commitments to patients involved round-the-clock steadfastness. See, for example, Harris (n.d.). Yet, if we recognize women physicians as struggling to balance career and family responsibilities, the issue is framed less accurately as 'lifestyle choices' and more as a negotiation of competing moral obligations connected with domestic life and career.

17 This project studied the effects of community-based education on dental students' sense of their ethical obligations to address the needs of the underserved. I conducted participant observation during required and voluntary service provision, and in five classes when students discussed these experiences; I also analyzed a sample (*n* = 216) of students' written reports on these experiences from between 1997 and 2006. I conducted semi-structured interviews with eleven students, seven clinic-based preceptors and staff, and eight faculty involved with community-based education; most of these were taped. All field notes and interviews were transcribed. Two faculty members and three students became key informants, offering me more extensive insights into their perspectives and experiences in the course of three years of research. Finally, I conducted a large group discussion with students and faculty on the topic of volunteering, which was taped and transcribed. All the names in this article are pseudonyms.

18 There are health professional education programs that do promote such obligations as cultural values, but these are the exception rather than the rule; see Davenport (2000) for one case study.

19 The national average of Medicaid reimbursement rates to dentists in 2008 reached only 60.5 percent of the rates paid by private insurers. Each state sets its own rates, with some as low as 30–50 percent of the dentists' so-called retail fees. Nor does Medicaid reimburse for all procedures. While the Early and Periodic Screening, Diagnostic and Treatment (EPSDT) benefit of Medicaid requires states to provide for the relief of pain and infections, and the restoration of teeth and maintenance of dental health for persons under age twenty-one, there are no federal requirements for states to cover any adult dental services. Most state Medicaid plans cover only emergency treatments, few offer comprehensive dental services to adults, and as states struggle to balance their budgets, many Medicaid plans have cancelled the minimal coverage for adult dental care previously provided. Clearly, the market place for oral healthcare in the USA is a highly stratified arena in which the vast majority of dentists serve the relatively affluent patients – while a minority serve the indigent and those on the public plan of Medicaid.

20 One example as to how they supposedly did this was through deliberately restoring only the caries visible to the naked eye, then taking X-rays and having to re-do them once more were diagnosed.

21 The ethical code of dentists does not include the norm of universal patient acceptance, and private practice dentists routinely limit their practices to patients who pay the costs they have established for their services (through direct payment or private insurance) (Peltier 2006). A study of North American dentists' interpretations of their 'social responsibility' found that the only obligations for treatment that all dentists agreed they had was to provide relief to a person in pain (Dharamsi et al. 2007).

22 In language that seems drawn straight from American-style management models, with their pay-for-performance metrics, the 2009 Russian Concept Statement for Health to the year 2020 (Ministerstvo 2009) discusses the need for patient outcomes and patient satisfaction measures to define 'quality' care. The Concept Statement also mentions the need for physician staff members of each institution to have self-governance – an important innovation that suggests transforming the power relations between administrators and clinicians, which speaks exactly to the kinds of issues regarding recognition and symbolic inclusion that I am emphasizing. Yet the brevity of this idea, and its uniqueness among the health policy documents I have analyzed, leads me to question the extent to which this innovation is being actively developed.

References

Antonova, N.L. (2007) 'Kachestvo meditsinskogo oblsuzhivaniia v sisteme obiazatel'nogo meditsinskogo strakhovaniia (na primere r. Ekaterinburga)', *SPERO*, 7: 191–98.

Bendina, O. (2009) 'Kuda ot etogo denesh'sia teper'': Normalizatsiia VICH-positivnykh zhenshchin meditsinskoi sistemoi', *Zhurnal Sotsiologii i Sotsial'noi Antropologii*, 1: 75–89.

Block, S.D., Clark-Chiarelli, N., Peters, A.S. and Singer, J.D. (1996) 'Academia's chilly climate for primary care', *JAMA*, 276: 677–82.

Curtis, S., Petukhova, N. and Taket, A. (1995) 'Health care reforms in Russia: the example of St Petersburg', *Social Science and Medicine*, 40(6): 755–65.

Davenport, B. (2000) 'Witnessing and the medical gaze: how medical students learn to see at a free clinic for the homeless', *Medical Anthropology Quarterly*, 14(3): 310–27.

Dharamsi, S., Pratt, D.D. and MacEntee, M.I. (2007) 'How dentists account for social responsibility: economic imperatives and professional obligations', *Journal of Dental Education*, 71(12): 1583–92.

Ebell, M. (2008) 'Future salary and US residency fill rate revisited', *JAMA*, 300(10): 1131–32.

Galarneau, C. (2011) 'Still missing: undocumented immigrants in health care reform', *Journal of Health Care for the Poor and Underserved*, 22(2): 422–28.

Goodman, D. (2008) 'Improving accountability for the public investment in health profession education: it's time to try health workforce planning', *JAMA*, 300(10): 1205–7.

Haden, N.K., Catalanotto, F.A., Alexander, C.J., Bailit, H., Battrell, A., Broussard Jr, J., Buchanan, J., Douglass, C.W., Fox III, C.E., Glassman, P., Lugo, R.I., George, M., Meyerowitz, C., Scott II, E.R., Yaple, N., Bresch, J., Gutman-Betts, Z., Luke, G.G., Moss, M., Sinkford, J.C., Weaver, R.G. and Valachovic, R.W. (2003) 'Improving the oral health status of all Americans: roles and responsibilities of academic dental institutions: the Report of the ADEA President's Commission', *Journal of Dental Education*, 67(5): 563–83.

Harris, R.R. (n.d.) *Dental Science in a New Age: A History of the National Institute of Dental Research.* www.usc.edu/hsc/dental/images_media/mobile_clinic_factsheet.pdf

Hauer, K.E., Durning, S.J., Kernan, W.N., Fagan, M.J., Mintz, M., O'Sullivan, P.S., Battistone, M., DeFer, T., Elnicki, T., Harrell, H., Reddy, S., Boscardin, C.K. and Schwartz, M.D. (2008) 'Factors associated with medical students' career choices regarding internal medicine', *JAMA*, 300(10): 1154–64.

Minkler, M. and Cole, T. (1997) 'Political and moral economy: getting to know one another', in M. Minkler, M. Meredith and C.L. Estes (eds) *Critical Gerontology: Perspectives from Political and Moral Economy*, Amityville, NY: Baywood Publishing Company.

Ministerstvo (2009) *Ministerstvo razvitiia sistemy zdravookhraneniia v Rossiiskoi Federatsii do 2020 g* [Russian Concept Statement for Health to the year 2020], Moscow: Ministerstvo zdravookhraneniia i sotsial'nogo razvitiia Rossiiskoi Federatsii. www. zdravo2020.ru/concept

Otto, M. (2007) 'For want of a dentist; Pr. George's boy dies after bacteria from tooth spread to brain', *The Washington Post*: B1.

Peltier, B. (2006) 'Codes and colleagues: is there support for universal patient acceptance?' *Journal of Dental Education*, 70(11): 1221–25.

Perlman, F., Balabanova, D. and McKee, M. (2009) 'An analysis of trends and determinants of health insurance and health care utilisation in the Russian population between 2000 and 2004: the "inverse care law' in action"', *BMC Health Services Research*, 9: 68, doi: 10.1186/1472-6963-9-68. www.biomedcentral.com/1472–6963/9/68

Rivkin-Fish, M. (2005) *Women's Health in Post-Soviet Russia: The Politics of Intervention*, Bloomington, IN: Indiana University Press.

——(2009) 'Tracing landscapes of the past in class subjectivity: practices of memory and distinction in marketizing Russia', *American Ethnologist*, 36(1): 163–79.

Rossiiskaia gazeta (2009) 'Zarplaty … salaries of doctors will rise in 2011', StartCapital, November 24. www.start-capital.ru

Rusinova, N.L. and Brown, J.V. (2003) 'Social inequality and strategies for getting medical care in post-Soviet Russia', *Health: An Interdisciplinary Journal for the Social Study of Health, Illness and Medicine*, 7(1): 51–71.

Shishkin, S.V., Bondarenko, N.V., Burdiak, A.I., Kel'manzon, K.M., Krasil'nikova, M.D., Popovich, L.D., Svetlichnaia, S.V., Selezneva, E.V., Sheiman, I.M. and

Shevskii, V.I. (2007) 'Analiz razlichii v dostupnosti meditsinskoi pomoshchi dlia naseleniia Rossii', Moscow: Independent Institute for Social Politics.

Tkatchenko-Schmidt, E., Atun, R., Wall, M., Tobi, P., Schmidt, J. and Renton, A. (2010) 'Why do health systems matter? Exploring links between health systems and HIV response: a case study from Russia', *Health Policy and Planning*, 25: 283–91.

Twigg, J. (2001) 'Russian health care reform at the regional level: status and impact', *Post-Soviet Geography and Economics*, 42(3): 202–19.

——(2002) 'Health care reform in Russia: a survey of head doctors and insurance administrators', *Social Science and Medicine*, 55: 2253–54.

United States Congress (2010) Patient Protection and Affordable Care Act. http://burgess.house.gov/UploadedFiles/hr3590_health_care_law_2010.pdf

4 Human oriented? Angels and monsters in China's health care reform[1]

Mei Zhan

Introduction

This chapter examines *yihuan guanxi*, or relations between medical professionals and patients, under China's health care reform. Invoking 'biopolitics' as a way of understanding the capillary workings of power in producing specific forms of lives and humans, I explore the ways in which different kinds of humans and tenuous claims to humanness are produced through the entanglement of government policy, market experimentation, and subject formation. Beginning in the mid-1990s, China's socialist health care system has been rapidly transformed into a set of highly marketized practices, institutions, products, and subjects. In recent years, even though the emphatically 'human-oriented' reform targets an emerging and heterogeneous middle-income citizenry as its primary subject and beneficiary, in everyday clinical encounters patients are confronted with rising health care costs, inefficiencies, and even unethical practices. Medical professionals meanwhile have come to bear the brunt of patients' frustration. No longer praised as the self-sacrificing 'angels' and 'heroes' of the socialist health care system, medical professionals are often portrayed in popular discourse as 'monsters in white coats' who epitomize the wrongs of the market and the failures of the reform. This chapter challenges such bifurcating representations of patients and doctors. Drawing on ethnographic and archival research, I suggest that, instead of being pitched against each other from the opposite ends of the spectrum of humanity, medical practitioners and patients alike strive after state-promoted middle-class dreams. Yet, marginalized in the human-oriented health care policy, the aspirations of medical professionals remain precarious and highly contested. Rather than wedged between patients and doctors, then, the friction in *yihuan guanxi* is produced from within situated discourses of the human, and thus must be understood within shifting understandings and practices of humanness.

Just human

Even before reaching the age of forty, Dr Han Xuemin was already an associate chief physician at one of the top biomedical hospitals in Shanghai.[2]

Being groomed for high-level hospital administration, he seemed on track for a blossoming career. Yet, when we sat down for a chat in the summer of 2009, Dr Han was rather anxious and deflated: 'Doctors work too hard. We are too tired. We don't make nearly as much money as people think. And nobody likes us – patients, the media, and even the Ministry of Health.' When asked to elaborate, he said, 'Our former Minister of Health called us "white-eyed wolves". This man had never worked at the patient's bedside, and knew nothing about our problems. It was only during the SARS outbreak (in 2003) that people all of a sudden remembered that we were "angels in white coats" and not monsters. But that was unnecessary. We are all humans and doctors want to be treated as humans just like everybody else.'

Zhang Wenkang is the said former Minister of Health who described the medical practitioner as a 'white-eyed wolf' or *baiyanlang* in Chinese, an expression for a greedy and ungrateful person devoid of conscience.[3] Even though Zhang's remark has earned him much animosity from health care workers, it reflects the popular perception of them as the personifications of the wrongs of China's experiments in health care reform, which, since the late 1990s, have quickly transformed health care from a public good provided by the state to a set of marketized and commodified practices, products, and institutions. As, in the eyes of the public, the profit-driven 'monsters in white coats' and 'butchers in white coats' come to replace life-saving 'angels' and selfless 'heroes', medical practitioners are often vilified when medical disputes arise, and are subjected to criticism, verbal abuse, and even physical violence from patients and their families. In a recent three-part survey on the 'state of survival' of doctors conducted by *Life Times* (*Shengming Shibao*), a popular newspaper on health care issues, 43 percent of doctors admit to having a 'love-and-fear' relationship with their profession, 98 percent complain about mental and emotional stress, and 80 percent pinpoint the greatest source of their stress in *yihuan guanxi*: the relations between medical practitioners and institutions on the one hand, and patients on the other (Liu and Wang 2008).

Strikingly, contentious discourses and manifestations of *yihuan guanxi* are intensifying at a time when governments at all levels begin to promote a 'human-oriented' (*yirenweiben*) approach to health care. This new approach, formalized at the Seventeenth National Congress of the Communist Party in October 2007, is intended to refocus health care on serving/servicing (*fuwu*) patients in order to correct the inequalities and inefficiencies brought upon by previous reform plans (Hu 2007; Chinese State Council 2009). However, the fact that the 'human' needs to be written into and fixed through official policy demonstrates the elusiveness of the human both in everyday clinical sociality, and in broader projects and processes of modernities and humanisms that shape the health care reform. It is noteworthy that the human turn is oriented specifically toward patients – referring primarily to so-called 'middle income' citizens – while medical practitioners remain unmentioned. Furthermore, the word *fuwu*, which straddles both 'serve' and 'service,' is poignantly ambiguous as it references both the socialist motto of 'serve the people' (*wei renmin fuwu*) and the more recent subsuming of health care under the 'service sector' (*fuwuxing hangye*) in postsocialist China's emerging and vibrant market economy. The position of medical practitioners in the human-oriented policy is thus both precarious and contradictory, with their humanness under construction and open to contestation.

Rather than being singularly and firmly wedged *between* patients and doctors, then, the incongruity and friction in *yihuan guanxi* are produced from *within* situated discourses of the human – the sociohistorical specificity of humanness, as well as the particular and often visceral relationships through which it is produced and enacted. A critical analysis of *yihuan guanxi* therefore cannot be built on the assumption that medical professionals and patients are pitched against each other from the opposite ends of the spectrum of humanity. In this chapter I propose that, instead of being entirely separate groups with irreconcilable interests, morals, and goals, medical practitioners and patients are deeply enmeshed in the 'biopolitics of the human,' by which I mean the sociohistorically situated fields of power and vexed intercorporeal relations through which different kinds of humans and particular claims to humanness are contingently produced, fiercely contested, and desperately recuperated. With a focus on the enmeshment of government policy, market experimentation, and humanism in its various articulations, I examine how medical practitioners in socialist and, especially, postsocialist China are configured as 'heroes', 'angels', 'monsters', and 'butchers in white coats': superhumans and subhumans in spite of their struggles to be 'just human'.

Particular biopolitics

Michel Foucault introduced the concept of biopolitics when discussing biopower, a distinctively modern and capillary form of power that suffuses each and every relationship, and produces human life itself as a distinctive subject of knowledge at once visible, knowable, and manageable. Revolutionary in its explications of the productive and discursive nature of knowledge, power, and politics, the Foucauldian conceptualization of biopolitics has generated lively discussions of governmentality and subject formation across national, geographic, and disciplinary boundaries. As the idea of biopolitics travels, it is important to keep in mind that it arises from specific sociohistorical conditions, and that part of the potency of this mode of analysis owes to its analytical specificity. First, Foucault (1980) located the emergence of biopolitics within the historical juncture between the *ancien régime* and the modern European state. 'Life as we know it' – compartmentalized within specific organisms and domains of knowledge, and in need of defending and regulating against the rest of the world – was unrecognizable until a mere 100 years ago (Cohen 2009; Helmreich 2009). Second, as noted by Gorgio Agamben (2009), Foucault's writings dealt with specific historical phenomena: prison, clinic, sexuality, asylum, and so forth. Yet his writings should not be – and have not been – read as historiographies or mere case studies: the material or phenomenon *is* itself theory, and the relation between phenomenon and theory is one that moves from particular to particular rather than from particular to general (Agamben 2009: 30). Instead of a theory of the general that provides a universal or global explanatory framework to account for particular ethnographic or historical phenomena, Foucault's work offers a methodology in and of the particular that enables us to uncover multiplicitous sites, acts, bodies, and relations of biopower, and to build specific analytics of biopolitics while resisting the impulse for analytical abstraction and transcendence.

In the case of *yihuan guanxi*, an analytic of biopolitics makes visible a complex web of discursive power relations where there are no easily identifiable victimizers and victimized, subjects and objects, powerful and powerless. The official media and public conversations in China routinely present patients as the underprivileged, the weak, and the victimized, and spare no efforts in detailing their sufferings. There is much less sympathy, in contrast, in the public sentiments and portrayals of medical practitioners. They are, simply put, the bad guys. Attentiveness to biopolitics, however, makes room for a critical analysis of the imbrications of government policy, market experimentation, and subjectification – an analysis that refrains from treating medical practitioners in the era of health care reform as mere instruments of the market or personifications of greed. My intention here is not to dismiss the suffering of patients or to take the side of the medical establishment: I am mindful of feminist critiques of dissolving the gritty materiality of power struggles into a field of the discursive and the rhetorical (Haraway 1991). I suggest instead that, in order to understand the complexity of *yihuan guanxi*, it is necessary to take into account not just structural power and violence, but also an assemblage of sociohistorically situated discourses, practices, and institutions of modernities and humanisms that constitute medical professionals as the embodied subjects that they are: in everyday clinical practice, and in everyday life more broadly speaking.

Furthermore, the analytical specificity of biopolitics allows us the space to imagine new and perhaps unfamiliar forms of life, knowledge, and politics beyond existing hegemonic paradigms. Over a decade of critical investigations into biopolitics in socialist and, especially, postsocialist China has laid bare how the state both reaches into and is constituted within the interstices of the most intimate aspects of everyday life – by regulating sexuality and reproduction, and by producing particular bodies and selves (e.g. Anagnost 1997; Rofel 1997, 2007; Farquhar 2002; Farquhar and Zhang 2005; Greenhalgh 2008). These discussions not only offer insights into the ways in which particular forms of life and ways of living emerge from the entwinement of socialism, marketization, liberalization, and globalization; more importantly, they keep in focus China's historical encounters with colonialism, modernity, and the Enlightenment narrative of history and progress – encounters that produce a spatiotemporality of lack-and-lag that continues to shape China's visions of the world and its place in it (Liu 1996; Karl 2002; Rofel 2007; Zhan 2009).

The 'otherness' of Chinese modernities, at once translocal and specific, is pivotal for understanding the ways in which the human is imagined and articulated through biopolitics in both socialist and postsocialist periods. Contemporary discussions of biopolitics in Europe and North America are often framed in reference to liberalized markets within which life is not only the subject of regulation, but also increasingly engineered by and subjected to the knowledge and logic of the market – in other words, life is becoming both an object and symptom of neoliberalism (e.g. Rose 1999). In celebratory popular and academic discourses about China, too, images of vibrant markets and enthusiastic mass consumption are invoked as tropes for China's transition from a production-based, planned economy toward economic liberalization and progress. Some are hopeful that China's new market economy, in producing enthusiastic consumer–subjects and cultivating horizontal relations of consumption, will create a more democratic everyday sociality similar to, if not identical with, European and North American liberal democracy (Davis 2000). Yet, as argued by a number of feminist scholars, an exclusive focus on subject formation within the market – as well as the assumption that the market is organized by a set of invisible laws and abstract logic – cannot fully account for the production of discrepant and embodied desires, interests, and subjects in everyday life that always exceed what is required by the function of the market (Tadiar 2004; Waldby and Mitchell 2006; Rofel 2007; Zhan 2005). The shift from socialism to postsocialism is therefore not a case of unidirectional transition toward neoliberalism (Wang 2004).[4] The discursively produced and inhabited human – and, more importantly, the right to be human – emerges not as a stable, self-explanatory point of reference for privatized social responsibilities or liberal humanistic discourses, but rather is relationally constituted and fiercely contested in everyday biopolitics and across discrepant sites.

Yihuan guanxi is such a set of everyday biopolitical interactions that requires a historicized analysis in which an account of the workings of the market is both indispensible and inadequate. In what follows, drawing on my field research in Shanghai and on discussions in Chinese media and internet forums, I explore the refiguration of the (in)humanness of patients, and especially medical practitioners, through doctor–patient relations: relations shaped both by the nostalgia and forgetting of knowledge production and practice of ethics in a socialist health care system that 'served the people,' and by experiences of the drastic transformation of health care into a set of marketized practices, products, and institutions expected to both serve *and* service the emergent 'middle-income' (*zhongceng shouru*) citizens.[5] Instead of producing the human through the logic of the market, the articulation of humanness in *yihuan guanxi* is both embodied and contradictory. On one hand, patients protest against being dehumanized in the commercialization of health care, and target medical practitioners as chief villains in the incompetent and sometimes inhumane treatment of patients. On the other, medical practitioners find themselves struggling to redefine their professional expertise and rethink professional ethics in a rapidly changing health care system molded by discrepant socialist and liberal humanist ideals that guide policy and market experimentations. Caught within conflicting visions of socialist and liberal humanisms, changing demands of market experimentations, and their own middle-class aspirations, medical practitioners are cast as 'angels' and 'monsters' whose humanness remains in the balance.

'Serve the people'

After the founding of the People's Republic of China in 1949, the Chinese government adopted a health care policy that prioritized preventing outbreaks of large-scale epidemics as well as meeting the basic health care needs of the masses, and especially the rural poor, who were amongst the staunchest supporters of the communist revolution.[6] Health care policy in the 1950s emphasized an orientation toward workers, peasants, and soldiers; focusing on prevention; promoting the solidarity between traditional Chinese and western medicines; and combining health care with socialist mass movement (Chen 2001; Scheid 2002; Taylor 2005; Zhan 2009). To this end, a low-cost and low-tech 'preventive medicine,' a mixture of biomedicine and traditional Chinese medicine, was invented and implemented across China and the rural areas in particular. Even today, retired and senior doctors of traditional Chinese medicine in Shanghai who participated in the 'clinic tours' (*xunhui yilaio*) in rural and suburban areas in the 1960s still recall the everyday medical practice of 'a bundle of needles (acupuncture), a handful of herbs [herbal medicine], and a pair of hands (*tuina*)'. In addition to practicing basic health care, doctors who obtained formal training in medical colleges in urban centers were encouraged to learn from peasants – especially the latter's practical medical knowledge that came out of agricultural work and class struggle. One senior practitioner of traditional Chinese medicine I interviewed fondly remembered spending hours biking from one village to another just to hear an old peasant woman talk about her own version of the 'five-element theory', a therapeutic principle and metaphor central to the understanding of body, illness, and healing in traditional Chinese medicine. 'That is the most insightful lecture on dialectics I have ever heard,' the practitioner told me.

As 'the people' (*renmin*) – or rather, the newly constituted proletariat masses and revolutionary subjects of the state – emerged as the primary subjects and beneficiaries of China's socialist health care system, they were also enlisted by the state to spearhead politicized health care campaigns that were part and parcel of China's socialist modernization. During the Great Leap Forward (1958–61), the Communist Party embarked on a project to collectivize and speed up China's industrial and agricultural production in order to 'catch up with Britain and overtake the United States' (*ganying chaomei*) within fifteen years (*People's Daily* 1958: 1). Armed with Marxist theory of labor and productivity, and taking to heart its historical materialism, the party leaders optimistically estimated that, by mobilizing China's vast reserve in manpower, the Chinese nation and its people would be able to bypass capitalism and reach communism within just decades (Liu 1958). The same optimism and the rush toward communist modernity ushered in highly politicized nationwide campaigns against infectious diseases and epidemics, now recast as matters of class struggle in which germs and diseases became just like 'class enemies'. One of the earliest and most famous campaigns was waged against schistosomiasis, a debilitating infectious disease borne by flukes living in water-dwelling snails in lakes, swamps, and rice paddies in the agricultural areas of southern China. Yujiang County, a rural county in Jiangxi Province, was singled out as an exemplar in the struggle against schistosomiasis. Armies of peasants and health care workers were mobilized to exterminate water snails. The eradication of schistosomiasis, incomplete as it later turned out to be, was hailed by Mao Zedong and the Communist Party as an unprecedented victory of the people in a political struggle against an epidemic that capitalist countries failed to vanquish (Chen and Liu 1958). In trying to 'catch up with' and 'overtake' capitalist countries, these health care campaigns both reproduced and subverted the temporality of lack-and-lag by attempting to 'jump' the order of history and progress.

In addition to high-profile health care campaigns, 'the people' and especially rural youths played a more mundane and indispensible role in China's health care system. Despite the presence of urban doctors who rotated their stays in rural areas, it was the 'barefoot doctors' (*chijiao yisheng*) who became front and center in the implementation and official representation of the socialist health care system (Farquhar 2002). Plucked from local communes, barefoot doctors practiced basic health care while at the same time being engaged in everyday agricultural production. Propaganda posters of barefoot doctors often depicted them carrying a medicine box, an agricultural tool, and a little red book of Chairman Mao's teachings. Omnipresent and larger than life, these selfless everyday socialist heroes who came from the people also typified how best to serve the people.[7]

China's people-centered health care system was hailed by the World Health Organization (WHO) as the model for all developing countries in the 1960s and 1970s for its success in providing affordable health care coverage for a large population and for its financial efficiency (Wang 2004). Its particular brand of socialist humanism and preventive medicine also became a trademark of Chinese medical teams that were sent to less developed countries in Africa, Latin America, and Southeast Asia as part of China's effort to forge and champion a racialized proletariat world during that period (Hutchison 1975; Snow 1988; Zhan 2009).[8] Among China's aid projects, medicine was the most successful because it was perceived as apolitical, in contrast to railway and dam constructions, and because it was desperately needed by the rural poor of developing countries.

However, even though the export of Chinese medical teams and the Chinese health care model was inspired by – and in turn globalized – the socialist vision of 'serve the people', this vision itself was animated by an international revolutionary consciousness fashioned out of racialized and class-girded understandings of the world (Zhan 2009). 'The people' was far from an all-encompassing concept of universal solidarity. Back home, and especially in urban centers, doctor–patient relations were shaped by the frictions between college-educated medical practitioners and the working-class masses they were asked to serve. During the Cultural Revolution (1966–76) in particular, medical practitioners and especially senior doctors were displaced from their positions in hospitals and clinics. Some were politically and physically persecuted. In Shanghai, a number of senior doctors who had played pivotal roles in founding state-run hospitals and medical colleges committed suicide as a consequence (Zhan 2009; also see Scheid 2002). Many of the less prominent doctors from the same generation found themselves in similar situations. Coming mostly from bourgeois and petit bourgeois families of intellectuals, merchants, clerks, and medical practitioners, and thus largely excluded from the proletariat masses, they felt alienated by the factory workers and Red Guards who ran the hospitals and clinics during those years. Some argued that their medical expertise suffered as they were either not allowed to practice medicine, or sent down to rural areas where only the most basic skills were required.

The experience of 'serve the people' was thus far from one of solidarity across geographic, professional, and class divides. On one hand, China's health care policy during the socialist period focused on the collective human produced through Marxist theory of labor, productivity, and class (albeit all with Chinese characteristics), postcolonial discourses of a racialized world, and modernist narratives of history and progress. This particular vision of the human promoted a populist and explicitly politicized approach to medical knowledge and expertise that problematized and marginalized the role of medical practitioners as the sole expert and authority in medical practices and clinical encounters. On the other hand, medical practitioners – especially with the addition of grassroots members such as the barefoot doctors – were called upon as heroic embodiments of socialist humanism in which the personal gave way to the collective.

Such ambiguities in 'serve the people,' however, are often lost on contemporary discourses of *yihuan guanxi*. Instead, ordinary citizens in China – including those who never actually lived through the socialist period – often invoke memories of state-planned and state-funded health care as the ideal model, in which health care was affordable, doctors were heroes and angels, and greed and selfishness were unheard of. Such romantic nostalgia is produced amidst increasing tensions between medical practitioners and patients in a marketized health care system, and in turn underscores the drastic transformation – or deterioration, as many of those in China would say – in both China's health care system and *yihuan guanxi* specifically. In order to understand medical professionals' drastic fall from grace, it is necessary to examine the twists and turns in China's health care policy and practice, and how, rather than serving the people, health care has become an ambiguous commodity in the 'service sector' of China's market economy.

Constructing the service sector

In 1992, Deng Xiaoping toured the southern cities Guangzhou, Shenzhen, and Zhuhai – part of China's first Special Economic Zone that spearheaded its economic reform and open-door policy. The ensuing period saw China intensify its economic reform and embark on the project of 'get on track with the world' (*yu shijie jiegui*). For many in China, Deng's speech during the tour signaled the beginning of a new push toward further market liberalization after the bloodshed of Tiananmen Square in 1989. Whereas China aimed at catching up with Britain and overtaking the United States during its rush toward communism in the 1950s, 'get on track with the world' articulated an altered modernist spatio-temporality in which late capitalist nation-states of North America and the European Union – as well as Australia and Japan – were at the center of China's worldly imaginary and its efforts to construct a 'moderately affluent society' (*xiaokang shehui*) (Zhan 2009). Rather than rural development and heavy industrial production, 'get on track with the world' emphasized turning urban areas, and especially coastal cities, into cosmopolitan centers of commerce, service, and consumption, and producing a substantive stratum of middle-income consumer-citizens as the mainstay of Chinese society and nation-state (Davis 2000; Zhang and Ong 2008).

As part of the project to get on track with the world, public goods such as health care, education, and housing became rapidly commodified to occupy a much bigger proportion of personal expenditure, more in line with consumption patterns in developed countries.[9] Preparations for health care reform began in the mid-1990s. Set in motion by the central government, the agenda of the health care reform was aimed at replacing state-funded health care coverage – which was deemed too much of a financial burden on the state and therefore unsustainable – with a system in which the citizen, their work unit, and the local government would share health care costs. In keeping the larger state project of marketization, hospitals and clinics became subsumed under the 'service sector' in China's emergent market economy.

Instead of drafting and implementing one reform plan across the country, however, selected urban areas and cities were chosen as sites for health care experimentation. Each was allowed to formulate its own experimental plan. In Shanghai, until 1998 the majority of permanent residents were placed under one of two health care plans: those in nonprofit public institutions and government agencies (e.g. schools and hospitals) were covered by 'public expense' (*gongfei*), which came directly from the municipal government; those in state-run enterprises (e.g. factories) were under 'work insurance' (*laobao*), funded by their work unit. Both were gradually phased out in the health care reform as individuals – whether working for nonprofit institutions, state-run enterprises, or the newly emerging private and/or foreign-owned sector – came to bear a much larger share of health care cost. The exact share of the cost borne by the individual varied depending on the specific draft of the experimental plans and the fiscal cycle. Between 1998 and 2010, there have been at least eight experimental plans – some publicized and some not, some implemented across the city and some only applied to specific age groups and professional occupations.[10]

In 1998, under the first city-wide health care reform plan, Shanghai's medical insurance would become financed primarily through contributions from local enterprises, including state-owned and collective-owned enterprises, joint ventures, foreign ventures, and private businesses. A Shanghai resident under employment was expected to pay a total premium of 7.5 percent of their monthly salary (Shanghai Medical Insurance Bureau 1998). Officials at the Shanghai Medical Insurance Bureau told me that the plan was conceived after they had toured various countries, including Germany, Singapore, and the United States, to observe and study their health care structures. First carried out among retirees on November 1, 1998, the plan caused a stir among various social groups and institutions. It favored the emerging class of white-collar workers, many of whom worked for well funded transnational and/or private companies. However, it added to the financial strains on workers in state-owned enterprises, whose income and job security were on the line as these enterprises experienced sharp declines in revenues and even bankruptcy during China's economic restructuring which, in urban centers in particular, saw heavy industries such as steel and textiles displaced by high-tech industries, finance, and the service sector.[11]

For hospitals and practitioners, too, health care reform, as well as market-ization more broadly speaking, presented unprecedented opportunities and challenges. A few entrepreneur-minded doctors began setting up their own clinics and manufacturing their own health products. More recently, private hospitals – some of which are foreign-owned and foreign-funded – began to compete with public hospitals in large cities. Yet, even for those who were successful in reinventing themselves during the reform, their new-found identity as practitioner–entrepreneurs was a troubling one. Li Fengyi, one of the most accomplished among them, insisted to me that his efforts at entre-preneurship allowed him to articulate his own health care visions – a new kind of holistic preventive medicine for middle-class urban dwellers – without having to deal with the bureaucracies at medical schools and hospitals. However, he was equally candid that he was running a business and was 'becoming more and more like a businessman'.

Those who did not become 'businessmen' faced even bigger challenges. At the Shanghai Shuguang Hospital of Traditional Chinese Medicine, a down-town hospital that served many elderly patients in the local communities, some regular patients came in to apologize to their doctors for not being able to continue treatment there. According to the health insurance plan of 1998, each individual was allowed to choose two hospitals to be covered by med-ical insurance: one neighborhood hospital and one district- or city-level hospital. Most patients chose biomedical hospitals for the second category, for fear of 'serious illnesses' that would require surgery and the latest bio-medical technologies and equipment. Even though hospital officials assured me that they did not see any noticeable drop in the volume of clinic visits or in-hospital patients after the commencement of the health care reform, doctors and nurses were equally adamant that they saw a remarkable drop in the body count of patients. Many expressed disgust at having to 'compete' for customers against other hospitals and clinics.[12] Many were confused about what their profession was all about. Dr Wang, a senior acupuncturist, blurted out aloud as she read a newspaper article on the health care reform: 'Are we part of the "service sector" (*fuwuxing hangye*) now? What does this mean? We are not pedicurists or restaurant servers: we treat illnesses and save lives!'

The health care reform thus entailed redefining the concept and the term *fuwu*: what counts as service, who is supposed perform it, and to whom it is oriented. Public goods for the masses no longer, medical practices and products were quickly turned into ambiguous commodities for a newly fashioned middle-income citizenry. It soon became obvious, however, that marketization did not bring financial efficiency or competitiveness as expected by the health care reform. In 2000, the WHO no longer advocated China's health care system as the model for all developing countries, and instead ranked it 188 on its scale of 'fairness in financial contribution' (Wang 2004: 18). In urban China, the privatization of health care and withdrawal of state subsidies has meant that, over a period of fifteen years between 1990 and 2004, whereas personal dispensable income rose by 5.24 times, health care expenditure increased by 19.57 times (Chinese Academy of Social Science 2007). Overall health care expenditure in 2005 amounted to 865.99 billion yuan, or 662.8 yuan (approximately $US86 in 2005) per capita (*Jiefang Ribao* 2007). Compared with 1981, the government's share of payment in 2005 dropped from 31.2 to 15.2 percent; society's share dropped from 42.6 to 26.5 percent; and the individual's share increased from 26.2 to 58.3 percent (*Jiefang Ribao* 2007).[13] All this prompted an official report from the National Reform and Development Commission, a special taskforce established by the Chinese State Council, to lament publicly that the Chinese health care system had 'contracted the American disease' of low efficiency and unfairness, and that the health care reform had been 'essentially unsuccessful' (Wang 2005). By the mid-2000s, 90 percent of the Chinese public were dissatisfied with the result of the health care reform (*Zhongguo Qingmanbao* 2005). Today, health care emerges as one of the biggest concerns for the middle-income Chinese citizens, as many complain about rising health care costs, worsening health care services and, especially, profit-seeking by medical practitioners at the expense of fulfilling their professional obligations of treating illnesses and saving lives.

The steadily increasing cases of medical disputes and scandals best illustrate the ways in which dissatisfactions are manifested in everyday clinical encounters. Heroes and angels no more, doctors and nurses today are often caricatured in everyday discourse as 'butchers in white coats.' Conjuring the image of patients as helpless animals awaiting wanton slaughtering, this metaphor works well in foregrounding the uneven power relations between medical practitioners and patients that threaten the bodily integrity, dignity, and embodied humanity of the patient. It accentuates the chasm between doctors and patients – to the point that they can be considered two different species across the human–animal divide. Yet it is not just the humanity of the patient that is under threat in the health care reform. Just as importantly, 'butchers in white coats' casts doctors and nurses as professional imposters whose precarious claim to humanity is clouded in shrouds of falsehood.

In what follows, I explore the rising medical disputes and scandals as an entry into the multiplicity and precariousness of the humanness of medical practitioners at the intersection of government policies, market experimentations, and discrepant articulations of the human. Even though representations of *yihuan guanxi* foreground the divide and even irreconcilability of patients and medical practitioners along the scale of humanness, I suggest instead that the incongruity lies within 'the human': not longer referring to the proletariat masses, the human is made continuous with the emerging and highly heterogeneous middle-income citizenry. The relation between medical practitioners and the definition of the new human is again a tenuous one. On one hand, they are expected to both serve and service the new humans – an expectation that only sharpens their image as the personification of the wrongs of the market. At the same time, as aspiring members of the middle-income citizenry themselves, medical practitioners are encouraged to live up to middle-class dreams, even though the requirements and constraints placed on them by changing government policies and market experimentations render these dreams nightmarish.

Recuperating the human

Since 2003, the government under President Hu Jintao has advocated a general approach of *yirenweiben* as its trademark policy. English translations of *yirenweiben* vary from 'putting people first', 'people oriented', 'human centered', to 'humanity as the base'. Some point out that 'human centered' is a term commonly used in business management in the United States. Like its contemporary English translations, the term's origin is also uncertain, pointing at both ancient Chinese and Greek philosophies. Some argue that the phrase derives from the Greek philosopher Protagoras' saying 'man is the measure of all things', which prioritizes the human in the order of all things and activities, including government policy. Meanwhile, some scholars argue that the exact term *yirenweiben* was first mentioned in the classic Chinese text *Guanzi*, compiled approximately between 725 and 645 BC. Attributed to Guan Zhong, the prime minister of the powerful Kingdom of Qi during the Spring and Autumn Period, the original text read: 'At the base of a powerful state are *ren* (*people* or *human*); if the base is in order then the state is strong; if the base is in disarray, the state is in danger.'[14]

Taken together, the origin story of *yirenweiben* indexes an effort to conjure a Chinese history of policy-making that prioritizes the people or the human, and a translocal outlook that emphasizes the congruence with Greek philosophy, which is central to a newly fabricated and yet increasingly global European intellectual history (Chakrabarty 2000). Today, the term not only characterizes policy-making by the central government in all aspects of its activities, but is also widely invoked in everyday discourses and especially market activities. A new catchphrase in advertisements and commercials, *yirenweiben* appears in efforts to sell a wide range of products ranging from environmentally conscious foods to more mundane commodities: *yirenweiben* recently appeared in a widely broadcast television commercial for the Nokia mobile phone. The term itself thus crystallizes the entanglement of policy-making and experiments in marketization: what happens in the central government, and what takes place in everyday life and market practice.

The latest master plan in health care reform has also promoted a human-oriented policy. First announced by President Hu Jintao in his Report to the Seventeenth National Congress of the Communist Party of China on October 15, 2007, a human-oriented health care policy would ensure that 'a reasonable and orderly pattern of income distribution will be basically in place, with middle-income people making up the majority and absolute poverty basically eliminated. Everyone will have access to basic medical and health services. The system of social management will be further improved' (Hu 2007).

After a year of intense discussion at various levels of the government, the human-oriented health care policy was formalized in an announcement from the State Council in 2009. An ostensible effort at combating the apparent dehumanizing effect of a marketized health care system, it makes explicit that the patient (*binren*) should be at the center of health care, and that the nature of health care as a public good needs to be restored (Chinese State Council 2009). The human-oriented health care policy, then, both recalls the agenda of the socialist health care system to serve the people, and subtly alters the scope of the people to put the middle-income citizenry front and center. However, this policy leaves the position of health care professionals rather ambiguous: as aspiring middle-income citizens, they are firmly within the embrace of the people and the human, and yet they are marginalized in a health care system re-centered around patients. Such ambiguities have profound manifestations in everyday clinical encounters, and especially in medical disputes and scandals in which medical practitioners are singled out as the embodiment of the greed of the market and ambiguous members of the emerging middle-income citizenry.

On July 28, 2010, a netizen self-named 'mutilated little chrysanthemum' posted on the website Tianya.cn that an obstetrics nurse at Phoenix Hospital in the city of Shenzhen, Guangdong Province stitched up her anus in retaliation for the patient's inability to present an adequate 'red envelope,' a euphemism for the cash gift contained inside.[15] Tianya being the largest internet forum in Chinese language, within a week the posting attracted more than 150,000 hits, 2000 responses, and half a dozen separate follow-up postings. Even before the incident could be substantiated, the netizens swiftly condemned the nurse and the hospital for their violation of the patient's body and abandonment of the most basic *yide* or medical ethics. Outcries against the 'inhumane' (*burendao*) treatment of the patient were rivaled only by denouncements of the 'inhuman' nurse (*bushiren*). Many posters stated as a matter of fact that medical practitioners no longer cared for anything except money. More disturbingly still, some argued that the nurse should have her own bodily orifices stitched up, be simply annihilated, or have her body torn to pieces by five horses – an ancient punishment reserved for the worst kind of criminals.

The incident drew instant attention from other popular Chinese websites, as well as local and provincial television stations and newspapers. Under pressure, the Shenzhen Committee of Healthcare and Birth Planning launched an investigation and organized a news conference within days. At the news conference, the obstetrics nurse wept as she insisted that she had only good intentions and was trying to 'tie up' a hemorrhoid that she discovered while delivering the baby, albeit without informing the patient or obtaining any authorization (Sina.com 2010). The general manager of the hospital, in addition, arranged a private meeting with the patient's husband to seek reconciliation. According to the husband, the manager lamented that the hospital staff had been irresponsible, and that the media had brought disaster upon the hospital. Punctuating his speech with bursts of tears, the general manager talked up his birthplace tie with the patient, and recounted his own record as a war hero by displaying his battle wounds from the China–Vietnam War of 1979 (Sina.com 2010).

The hospital suspended the nurse for performing surgical procedure without the required expertise or qualification, and for soliciting a red envelope. The results of the official investigation by the police and various medical experts, however, came out 'inconclusive' as they disagreed with each other regarding which procedure was actually performed and whether it was necessary, thus drawing further criticisms from the patient's family, the netizens, and the media. Strikingly, the *People's Daily*, the official newspaper of the Chinese party-state, joined the discussion, with three editorials within a week. Noting that patients are the weak group (*ruoshi qunti*) in *yihuan guanxi*, one editorial in particular argued that such inequality is the consequence of asymmetrical expertise and information dissemination as well as the destruction of medical ethics by 'a few' profit-seeking practitioners (Miao 2010). Citing the Chinese saying that 'being in a different profession is like being on the other side of the mountain,' the *People's Daily* editorial urged the media to deepen their 'medical knowledge' when reporting medical disputes so as to mediate and enhance mutual trust between medical professionals and patients (Miao 2010).

The 'stitched anus incident,' as it is nicknamed, is only the latest in the festering medical disputes and scandals and of increasingly contentious *yihuan guanxi*. The not-so-subtle identification with the lower opening of the digestive system and its mutilation captures the gritty 'intercorporeality' (Waldby

2002; Weiss 1999) of a health care system on a dramatic descent into a bottomless pit of dysfunction and immorality. With accusations of medical wrongdoing on the rise, medical practitioners in urban China today work in constant fear of disgruntled patients 'making trouble' (*naoshi*), ranging from obstructing everyday operations at clinics and hospitals, mounting legal challenges, public humiliation of doctors and nurses, destruction of hospital properties, to the beating and even murder of medical professionals. A survey by the Chinese Ministry of Health shows that 70 percent of health care professionals have received threats from disgruntled patients (Sina.com 2005). When a practitioner of traditional Chinese medicine renowned for both his medical skills (*yishu*) and his medical ethics (*yide*) was hacked down by an angry patient in broad daylight in 2005, an overwhelming majority of the general public were sympathetic and even supportive of the murderer (Xilu.com 2005).

In spite of increasing cases of violence and violent sentiments against medical practitioners, official and public discourses converge on the view that health care reform has reduced patients to reluctant consumers and disempowered objects of commercial-medical practices; at the same time, medical practitioners have come to personify the greed of a profit-driven health care system becoming increasingly unethical and even inhuman(e) in its treatment of patients. Compelling expressions of widespread discontent with the health care *status quo*, these oppositional discourses of *yihuan guanxi* define the inequality in doctor–patient relations within the parameters of the market, especially in terms of the uneven possession of, and access to, expert knowledge, as well as radically different investments in medical ethics. However, in presenting medical professionals as the all-powerful culprits, they tend to present the image of a market that works by its own inherent logic of profit-making, and an impoverished understanding of the humanness of doctors and nurses as no more than the personifications of the market. The construction of a pure market thus obscures the complex field of power that shapes the mutual imbrications of practitioners and patients in biopolitical discourses of medical expertise and ethics through which different kinds of bodies and humans are constituted, and where claims to humanness are staked.

To begin, medical disputes take place within often mundane, sometimes intense, and always intercorporeal clinical and hospital encounters and interactions. Many patients I interviewed related to me that they understand perfectly well that doctors and nurses work hard, need to support their families, buy apartments, send their children to school, and take care of aging parents – just like the patients themselves. However, such sentiments quickly give way to frustration and accusations of bad conscience when specific medical encounters are concerned. As one patient put it,

> It is hard to go into a hospital, wait in a long line, pay a lot of money, and still have the doctors and nurses treat you very coldly and harshly. And you have to give them red envelopes if you have a serious illness. Then you wonder if they give you a particular prescription or

recommend a procedure because it is necessary, or because they get more kickbacks from it. You hear so many horror stories and you just can't trust them anymore.

It is much easier, then, to relate to medical practitioners through shared middle-class ideals and problems, than in particular intercorporeal encounters where personal and bodily stakes are high, and where 'trust' over both medical expertise and medical ethics are at best uncertain. It is noteworthy that, even though the *People's Daily* editorial framed the dispute over the 'stitched anus incident' in terms of insurmountable barriers between patients and medical practitioners in professional knowledge and expertise, the possession of, and access to, medical knowledge in everyday discourse and practice is far less clear cut. As part of the socialist legacy in which practical medical knowledge was valued, many patients have some knowledge and understanding about basic health care and are not afraid to voice their own opinions when facing doctors and nurses. This is particularly problematic for the clinical practice of traditional Chinese medicine, where doctors are routinely challenged by patients over prescriptions and treatments, especially when it comes to emergency care, for which Chinese medicine is often considered less effective compared with biomedicine. Doctors express fear over giving herbal remedies instead of performing standard biomedical procedures and prescribing antibiotics. As Doctor Tang, a chief physician at Shuguang Hospital, put it:

> I have confidence in traditional Chinese medicine. But when a patient comes in with a cold, I prescribe antibiotics as they would always expect me to do. If I give patients herbs and they do not get better, they would be angry because I did not prescribe antibiotics. It has nothing to do with whether I am right or wrong in terms of treatment. But you must understand that I do not want any trouble with patients: I don't want them to complain to the hospital administration or beat me up.

The mistrust between medical practitioners and patients is thus not easily reduced to a matter of professional barriers, and the solution therefore cannot lie in 'communication' alone: not only do patients to a certain extent share medical knowledge with practitioners, but the professional expertise within medical discourses is heterogeneous, uneven, and open to contestation. It is precisely the sharedness of knowledge, as well as the unevenness within the medical profession, that enables patients to challenge the authority of medical practitioners in everyday clinical socialities and face-to-face interactions.

Furthermore, the rise in medical disputes and scandals is not just the byproduct of fraught clinical encounters, but also needs to be understood in relation to larger experiments in marketization, in which the state plays an active role, and where heterogeneous desires, interests, and financial practices always exceed the 'logic' of the market. Many of those who voice their anger at the medical professionals in the 'stitched anus incident,' for example, also concede begrudgingly that, even though this particular incident was extreme, giving a red envelope to doctors, anesthesiologists, nurses, and whoever else in charge has become all but expected.[16] Some recount their own experiences of negligence and abuse at the hands of medical professionals after failing to meet the informal and yet expected 'market price' of their service. In Shanghai, it is common knowledge that a red envelope ranges anywhere between 2000 and 10,000 yuan, depending on the type and seriousness of the illness as well as the seniority and professional reputation of the doctor in charge. In addition, the red envelope is not only for the doctor, but also for nurses, anesthesiologists, and whoever else is involved in the care of the patient. When discussing the practice of giving red envelopes, most patients say they dislike the practice, but also admit to being 'relieved' when the medical practitioners take their offer: a sign that patients can feel more 'assured' that they will be taken care of. Some suggest that they are only paying the 'real price' of a doctor's service, as it goes straight to the practitioner. Many doctors and nurses, on the other hand, admit to accepting red envelopes, though they are not proud of it. Some argue that there is nothing wrong with accepting a red envelope as long as they do not actively seek it, or mistreat the patient when no red envelope is given.

The general sentiment is that doctors and nurses work harder than many other professionals, deal with a high level of stress, and are underpaid compared with other college-educated professionals. Among the 2183 doctors surveyed from eight cities in the aforementioned three-part survey conducted by *Life Times*, 80 percent work between 8 and 12 hours a day and do not have time to drink water during a work day; 67 percent work continuously over 36 hours; 83 percent have colleagues who suffer from cancer; and 37 percent have colleagues who had 'sudden death' (Jiang et al. 2008). 'Sudden death' in particular is an increasingly common cause of death among urban white collar workers as the consequence of stressful work and living situations (Zhan 2009). The same survey reveals that 75 percent of doctors say that their annual salary is under 40,000 yuan (approximately $US5900), and 83 percent are unhappy with their income (Liu 2008). In Shanghai, 18 percent of a 'middle-income' resident's pay goes to social security (8 percent), medical insurance (2 percent), unemployment insurance (1 percent), and the public housing fund (7 percent) – leaving 'far from enough', in the words of many doctors, for other expenses including childcare, tuition, and housing payments. As one doctor put it during a conversation with me: 'if I really want to make money I would have changed my profession already. My classmates from medical school who now work as representatives for pharmaceutical companies are much better paid. But I am still here because I believe in what I do.'

Rather than fitting readily into the category of corruption and bribery, then, the red envelope is often an informal, if controversial, market practice that not only makes a particular clinical encounter work, but also provides partial assurance of qualified 'trust' between medical practitioners and patients – albeit at a price. The dispute and interest generated by the 'stitched anus incident' are not about the practice of giving red envelopes *per se*, but are about the *terms* of these transactions as well as questions of accountability: what is fair, who gets to set the price, and who bears the consequence (and what kind of consequence) when transactions and relations break down. On one hand, distressed by the medical practitioner's mutilation of her body, the patient and her husband seek to reclaim her dignity and humanity expressed through the right to bodily integrity and ethical health care. On the other, in recounting his life story and baring his own scarred body, the hospital manager attempts to conjure the common memory of a socialist past in which self-sacrificial heroism was imaginable and a shared and embodied humanity was within reach. Yet, tangled up in market and clinical encounters, the humanness of both patients and medical practitioners remains mutilated at best: an aspiration rather than actuality.

Conclusions

Medical practitioners in China are entangled in ambiguous and incongruous biopolitics of *yihuan guanxi*, in which their very claims to being human are at stake. Rather than the embodiments of either socialist ideals or the ills of the market, the humanness – or, rather, inhumanness – of medical practitioners always exceeds the laws of the market and the command of state policy. Discourses of middle-classness set the terms for the humanity of medical practitioners, both at work and in leisure and life. However, rather than unifying what it means to be human, these discourses are invoked and deployed in divergent and contradictory ways at the intersection of policy-making, market experimentation, and everyday subject formation. Suspended in the seemingly irreconcilable ideals of the selfless socialist hero and the maximizing creature of the market, these medical practitioners are always on the verge of falling into the abyss of being subhuman. Far from a ready-made and universalistic human subject, the medical practitioner is always in the process of (un)becoming.

What does this mean for understanding biopolitics in and of postsocialist China? Rather than a 'multiplication of contexts' (Andrews 1996), in which China is a particular case of – or anomaly in – global neoliberal formation of the human, the rise and the predicament of the 'middle class' in China offers an analytical opportunity for us to re-examine some of the most basic assumptions about what it means to be a medical practitioner, what it means to be a patient, what it means to be an entrepreneur or consumer – and what it means and takes to be *somewhat* human.

Notes

1 This chapter grew out of a paper presented at the Society for the Social Studies of Science Annual Meeting in 2009. It has appeared in a similar form in *East Asian Science, Technology and Society* 5(3) (2011): 291–311. I am grateful for funding support from the Center for East Asian Studies and the Center for Global Peace and Conflict Studies at the University of California, Irvine.

2 I use pseudonyms throughout the text to protect my interlocutors' identities.

3 Ironically, Zhang's tenure of five years ended in spring 2003, when he was removed from the post for mishandling the SARS epidemic, during which the reputation of medical professionals was briefly restored (Zhan 2008).

4 For comparisons with other 'postsocialist' states, see discussions of health care reform in Russia by Michele R. Rivkin-Fish (2005), and in Poland by Peggy Watson (2006; 2011). Both take into account – and also challenge – the framing of such health care reforms in terms of individualization and liberalization. Importantly, these authors explicate the refigurations of postsocialist societies in terms of social, economic, and gender inequalities. Watson (2011), in particular, argues that health care reforms and liberalizations in postsocialist states must be understood in transnational, national, and local power relations and fields.

5 The official discourses in China most regularly use the term 'middle income' rather than 'middle class.'

6 See Ann Anagnost (1997) for an insightful discussion of the ways in which various local social problems and conflicts in rural China at the time were translated and transformed through communist government campaigns and Marxist theory into 'class struggles' – thereby inventing a unified rural proletariat class.

7 See Farquhar (2002) for an insightful discussion of the people's hero Lei Feng, a key symbol of selfless socialist heroes who epitomized how to 'serve the people'.

8 When receiving an African delegation, Mao famously said that 'race problem is class problem' and that 'we blacks must stick together' (Zhan 2009).

9 Like health care, education and housing (real-estate ownership) have also become major sources of complaints in China today. See Zhang (2010) for more discussions of the real-estate market and the rise of new social statuses associated with real-estate ownership.

10 As of 2010, a resident of average income is required to contribute 2 percent of their income.

11 The late 1990s witnessed a wave of 'stepping down the post' (*xiagang*) among factory workers. In Shanghai, textile factory and steel factory workers – nicknamed 'Big Brother Steel' and 'Big Sister-in-law Textile' – bore the brunt of the *xiagang* wave.

12 Given the precarious position of traditional Chinese medicine within China's health care system, and especially in relation to biomedicine, marketization opened up another site where traditional Chinese medicine had to wrestle with biomedicine – not only over medical knowledge and authority, but also over the bodies of consumer–patients themselves.

13 'Society' here includes various enterprises, bureaucratic and other nonprofit institutions, and neighbourhood communities.

14 '夫霸王之所始也，以人为本。本理则国固，本乱则国危。' This is taken from the second page of *Guanzi*, Vol. II, published by Shangwu Yinshuguan in 1936. I leave the translation of 'ren' (人) deliberately ambiguous here because in classical Chinese 'min' (民) is usually used specifically to refer to 'people' who are the subjects of the state even though the contemporary Chinese term for 'people' consists of both 'ren' and 'min' (人民).

15 'Netizen' is the common English translation of *wangmin*, which literally means 'people of the internet'. Whereas the Chinese phrase places emphasis on *min* or 'people', which in classic Chinese references the governed subjects, its English translation plays off the word 'citizen' and is oriented toward an alternative form of participatory citizenship.

16 See Rivkin-Fish's (2005) account of cash-gift giving in postsocialist Russia. Rivkin-Fish argues that rather than 'briberies', these payments are now informal monetary exchanges that are part and parcel of shifting Russian economy and sociality.

References

Agamben, G. (2009) *The Signature of All Things: On Method*, transl. Luca D'Isanto with Kevin Attell, New York: Zone.

Anagnost, A. (1997) *National Past-Times: Narrative, Representation, and Power in Modern China*, Durham, NC: Duke University Press.

Andrews, B. (1996) *The Making of Modern Chinese Medicine, 1895–1937*, PhD thesis, University of Cambridge.

Chakrabarty, D. (2000) *Provincializing Europe: Postcolonial Thought and Historical Difference*, Princeton, NJ: Princeton University Press.

Chen, B.Y. and Liu, G.H. (1958) 'Diyimian Hongqi—Ji Jiangxi Yujiangxian Genben Xiaomie Xuexichongbing de Jingguo' [The first red flag: the process of how schistosomiasis was completely annihilated in Yujiang County, Jiangxi Province], Xinhua News Agency, June 29.

Chen, N. N. (2001) 'Health, wealth, and the good life', in *China Urban: Ethographies of Contemporary Culture*, N.N. Chen, C.D. Clark, S.Z. Gottschang and L. Jeffery (eds), Durham, NC: Duke University Press.

Chinese Academy of Social Science (2007) *Shenhui Baozhang Lüpishu* [Social Security Green Book], Beijing: Chinese Academy of Social Sciences.

Chinese State Council (2009) *Guowuyuan Guanyu Yinfa Yiyao Weisheng Tizhi Gaige Jinqi Zhongdian Shishi Fangan (2009–2011) de Tongzhi* [The State Council's notice regarding printing emphases to be implemented in the healthcare reform in the near future, 2009–11], Announcement 2009, No. 12.

Cohen, E. (2009) *A Body Worth Defending: Immunity, Biopolitics, and the Apotheosis of the Modern Body*, Durham, NC: Duke University Press.

Davis, D.S. (2000) 'Introduction: A revolution in consumption', in D.S. Davis (ed.) *The Consumer Revolution in Urban China*, Berkeley, CA: University of California Press.

Farquhar, J. (2002) *Appetites: Food and Sex in Post-Socialist China*, Durham, NC: Duke University Press.

Farquhar, J. and Zhang, Q. (2005) 'Biopolitical Beijing: pleasure, sovereignty, and self-cultivation in China's capital', *Cultural Anthropology*, 20(3): 303–27.

Foucault, M. (1980) *History of Sexuality*, Vol. I, New York: Vintage Books.

Greenhalgh, S. (2008) *Just One Child: Science and Policy in Deng's China*, Berkeley, CA: University of California Press.

Guan, Z. (1936) *Guanzi*, Vol. 2, Shanghai: Shangwu Yinshuguan [Shangwu Publishing House].

Haraway, D. (1991) *Simians, Cyborgs, and Women: the Reinvention of Nature*, New York: Routledge.

Helmreich, S. (2009) *Alien Ocean: Anthropological Voyages into Microbial Seas*, Princeton, NJ: Princeton University Press.

Hu, J.T. (2007) *Hold High The Great Banner of Socialism with Chinese Characteristics and Strive for New Victories in Building a Moderately Prosperous Society in all Respects*, Report to the Seventeenth National Congress of the Communist Party of China, October 15, 2007.

Hutchison, A. (1975) *China's African Revolution*, London: Hutchinson.

Jiang, N.Q., Yang, L.C. and Liu, J.J. (2008) 'Yisheng Daodi You Duolei' [How tired are doctors?], Investigation Series on the State of Survival of Doctors in China, Part 2, *Shengming Shibao* [*Life Times*], March 11.

Jiefang Ribao (2007) 'Yigai: Ruhe Pingheng Gongping Yu Xiaolü?' [Healthcare reform: how to balance fairness and efficiency], *Jiefang Ribao* [*Jiefang Daily*], May 20.

Karl, R. (2002) *Staging the World: Chinese Nationalism at the Turn of the Twentieth Century*, Durham, NC: Duke University Press.

Liu, J.J. (2008) 'Yisheng De Shouru Dibudi' [Is a doctor's income low?], Investigation Series on the State of Survival of Doctors in China, Part 3, *Shengming Shibao* [*Life Times*], March 18.

Liu, J.J. and Wang, X. (2008) 'Baixing Ruhe Pingshuo Yisheng' [How do ordinary people evaluate doctors?], Investigation Series on the State of Survival of Doctors in China, Part 1, *Shengming Shibao* [*Life Times*], March 4.

Liu, L.H. (1996) *Translingual Practice: Literature, National Culture, and Translated Modernity—China, 1900–1937*, Stanford, CA: Stanford University Press.

Liu, S.Q. (1958) 'Editorial', *Beijing Ribao* [*Beijing Daily*], June 30.

Miao, M. (2010) 'Yihuan You Jiufen, Meiti Yao Lengjing' [The media need to remain cool-headed when facing disputes between medical practitioners and patients], *People's Daily*, August 3: 14.

People's Daily (1958) 'Editorial', *People's Daily*, January 1.

Rivkin-Fish, M. (2005) *Women's Health in Post-Soviet Russia: the Politics of Intervention*, Bloomington, IN: Indiana University Press.

Rofel, L. (2007) *Desiring China: Experiments in Neoliberalism, Sexuality, and Public Culture*, Durham, NC: Duke University Press.

——(1997) *Other Modernities: Gendered Yearnings in China after Socialism*, Berkeley, CA: University of California Press.

Rose, N. (1999) *Powers of Freedom: Reframing Political Thought*, Cambridge: Cambridge University Press.

Scheid, V. (2002) *Chinese Medicine in Contemporary China: Plurality and Synthesis*, Durham, NC: Duke University Press.

Shanghai Medical Insurance Bureau (1998) *Medical Insurance System Reform in Shangha*, Shanghai: Shanghai Medical Insurance Bureau.

Sina.com (2005) 'Qicheng Yiwu Renyuan Ceng Shou Weixie' [Seventy per cent of medical professionals have received threats].

——(2010) 'Shenzhen Chanfu "Bei Feng Gangmen An" Diaochao' [Investigation into the case of a new mother's 'stitched anus' in Shenzhen]. http://news.sina.com.cn/s/sd/2010-08-05/112620832618.shtml

Snow, P. (1988) *The Star Raft: China's Encounter with Africa*, London: Weidenfeld and Nicolson.

Tadiar, N. (2004) *Fantasy Production: Sexual Economies and Other Philippine Consequences for the New World Order*, Hong Kong: Hong Kong University Press.

Taylor, K. (2005) *Chinese Medicine in Early Communist China, 1945–63: A Medicine of Revolution*, New York: RoutledgeCurzon.

Tianya.cn (2010) *Yin Mei Zhunbeihao Hongbao, Shenzhen Fenghuang Yiyuan De Zhuchanshi Jinran Ba Wode Gangmen Fengshang Le* [The obstetrics nurse at Shenzhen Fenghuang Hospital stitched up my anus because I did not prepare a proper red envelope], Tianya.cn. www.tianya.cn/publicforum/content/free/1/1949303.shtml

Waldby, C. (2002) 'Biomedicine, tissue transfer and intercorporeality', *Feminist Theory*, 3(3): 239–54.

Waldby, C. and Mitchell, R. (2006) *Tissue Economies: Blood, Organs, and Cell Lines in Late Capitalism*, Durham, NC: Duke University Press.

Wang, J. (2005) 'Guowuyuan Yanjiujigou Chen Woguo Yigai Gongzuo Jiben Buchenggong' [Research institution of the State Council declares that our country's healthcare reform is essentially unsuccessful], *Zhongguo Qingnianbao* [*China Youth Daily*], July 28.

Wang, S. (2004) 'China's health system: from crisis to opportunity', *Yale-China Health Journal*, 3: 5–49.

Watson, P. (2011) 'Fighting for life: health care and democracy in capitalist Poland', *Critical Social Policy*, 31: 53–76.

——(2006) 'Unequalizing citizenship: the politics of Poland's health care change', *Sociology*, 40: 1079–96.

Weiss, G. (1999) *Body Images: Embodiment as Intercorporeality*, London and New York: Routledge.

Xilu.com (2005) 'Yige Mingyi De Si He Ta Chengshou De Tuoma [A famous doctor's death and the condemnations he endured], http://bbs15.xilu.com/cgi-bon/bbs/view news?forum=qzll& message=2423

Zhan, M. (2005) 'Civet cats, fried grasshoppers, and David Beckham's pajamas: unruly bodies after SARS', *American Anthropologist*, 107(1): 31–42.

——(2008) 'Wild consumption: privatizing responsibilities in the time of SARS', in L. Zhang and A. Ong (eds) *Privatizing China*, Ithaca: Cornell University Press.

——(2009) *Other-Worldly: Making Chinese Medicine through Transnational Frames*, Durham, NC: Duke University Press.

Zhang, L. (2010) *In Search of Paradise: Middle-class Living in a Chinese Metropolis*, Ithaca, NY: Cornell University Press.

Zhang, L. and Ong, A. (eds) (2008) *Privatizing China: Socialism from Afar*, Ithaca, NY: Cornell University Press.

Zhongguo Qingnianbao (2005) 'Zhongguo Jiucheng Gongzhong Buman Shinian Lai Yiliao Tizhi Gaige Fangmian Bianhua' [Ninety per cent of China's public are dissatisfied with ten years of changes in healthcare reform], *Zhongguo Qingnianbao* [*China Youth Daily*], August 11: 1.

5 We are all in this together – European policies and health systems change

Meri Koivusalo

Introduction

The European Union (the EU) was initially established, and the Treaty of Rome signed, in 1957 (see Box 5.1). The Treaty of Rome was based on common markets and economic cooperation between Member States, but it also included health care-related commitments, such as coordination among Member States with respect to social security and occupational health and safety. However, for a long time the influence of European policies on national health care systems was limited, if in practice almost non-existent. One example of this is the fact that when Finland, Sweden and Austria joined the EU in 1995, it was wrongly understood in Finland that there would be no impact on health and social services. Indeed, this was what was claimed by decision-makers. If the electorate had thought otherwise, it could have changed the result of the vote on joining the EU. Health implications of the EU were considered predominantly in the context of public health policies; for example, when Finland and Sweden joined the EU, they negotiated time frames before border measures were fully lifted from alcohol products.

> **Box 5.1. European Union: background and powers**
>
> In the aftermath of the Second World War, in 1949, the West European nations established the Council of Europe, which still functions.
>
> The EU has its background in further integration sought by six nations (Belgium, France, Germany, Italy, Luxembourg and the Netherlands), which took further steps towards European integration in the context of the European Coal and Steel Community (ECSC), subscribing to the Schuman declaration in 1950.
>
> In 1951, these countries signed the Treaty of Paris establishing the ECSC. This Treaty is important as it foresees the establishment of key European institutions, including the Court of Justice, Parliament, Council of National Ministers and Executive Council. The Treaty of Rome was signed in 1957, consisting of treaties establishing the

European Economic Community (EEC) and the European Atomic Energy Community (Euratom). The UK, Denmark and Ireland joined the European Community in 1973, Greece in 1981, and Spain and Portugal in 1986. Finland, Sweden and Austria joined in 1995; Hungary, the Czech Republic, Slovakia, Slovenia, Estonia, Lithuania, Latvia, Malta, Cyprus and Poland joined in 2004; and Bulgaria and Romania in 2007. The current EU thus consists of twenty-seven Member States.

The EU's governance is based on negotiated treaties, which lay down the basis for further collaboration and integration. The key treaties are:

- Treaty of Rome, 1957

    - established economic cooperation and the European Economic Community

- Treaty of Maastricht, 1992

    - created the EU and led to the creation of the single currency (euro)

- Treaty of Amsterdam, 1997

    - established the basis for a common foreign and security policy

- Treaty of Nice, 2001

    - made eastward expansion possible

- Treaty of Lisbon, 2007

    - initially amended the treaties of Rome and Maastricht under a treaty establishing a constitution for Europe, which was not accepted by French and Dutch voters in 2005. A slightly amended version was signed in Lisbon in 2007.

The **European Court of Justice** is important due to its role in interpretations and judgements with respect to disputes over Treaty provisions.

The **European Commission** in practice forms the executive and civil service, with responsibility for taking commitments further as well as the right to initiate new policies.

While the powers of the **European Parliament** have been increased through treaty negotiations, the main role of the Parliament is in scrutinising, following and amending policies and legislation proposed by the Commission. The European Parliament is the only directly elected body in the EU, and currently consists of 736 Members of the European Parliament.

The **European Council** (or Council of the European Union) is governed by Member States' national ministries. It essentially mediates the voice of elected Member State governments in European policy-making, legislative and policy proposals by the Commission. The practice of co-decision that applies to most of the decisions in the EU in practice implies that Parliament and Council must both agree to initial proposals made by the Commission for them to proceed.

More information on the EU is available at www.europa.eu

The Finnish 'newcomers" anticipation that joining the EU would have no influence on national health policies reflects well the situation that existed in the mid-1990s, when different types of health systems, based on different principles, coexisted with little interference from the EU. The Maastricht Treaty and the commitment to internal markets, as well as the establishment of the European Monetary Union (EMU), have been seen as crucial moments for European welfare states; nevertheless, these were – again – not expected to have substantial practical implications for health systems.

In EU governance, the European Commission has the right to initiate policies, whereas the European Council, which is governed by Member States, and the European Parliament, which is voted in by European citizens, can only encourage, amend or delay further development of the policy process (see Box 5.1). However, the broader legal framework and basis for the legitimacy of EU action is defined by negotiated treaties. The European Court of Justice interprets and provides guidance with respect to treaty articles and provisions. The European Commission has traditionally maintained complementary powers and competence in public health. However the adoption of the Lisbon Treaty extended the competence of the European Commission, giving it precedence over Member State legislation in areas of 'shared' competence (see Box 5.2).

Box 5.2. The Lisbon Treaty

The Lisbon Treaty negotiated changes in the consolidated Treaty on the Functioning of the European Union, with Articles 2, 3 and 4 defining competences (key provisions are indicated in bold by the author).

Article 2

1. When the Treaties confer exclusive competence on the Union in a specific area, only the Union may legislate and adopt legally binding acts, the Member States being able to do so themselves only if so empowered by the Union or for the implementation Union acts.
2. When the Treaties confer on the Union a competence shared with the Member States in a specific area, the Union and the Member States may legislate and adopt legally binding acts in that area. The

Member States shall exercise their competence to the extent that the Union has not exercised its competence. **The Member States shall again exercise their competence to the extent that the Union has decided to cease exercising its competence.**
... / ...

5. In certain areas and under the conditions laid down in the Treaties, the Union shall have competence to carry out actions to support, coordinate or supplement the actions of the Member States, without thereby superseding their competence in these areas.

Article 3

1. The Union shall have exclusive competence in the following areas:

   (a) customs union;
   (b) **the establishing of the competition rules necessary for the functioning of the internal market;**
   (c) monetary policy for the Member States whose currency is the euro;
   (d) the conservation of marine biological resources under the common fisheries policy;
   (e) **common commercial policy.**

2. The Union shall also have exclusive competence for the conclusion of an international agreement when its conclusion is provided for in a legislative act of the Union or is necessary to enable the Union to exercise its internal competence, or in so far as its conclusion may affect common rules or alter their scope.

Article 4

1. The Union shall share competence with the Member States where the Treaties confer on it a competence which does not relate to the areas referred to in Articles 3 and 6.

2. Shared competence between the Union and the Member States applies in the following principal areas:

   (a) **internal market;**
   (b) social policy, for the aspects defined in this Treaty;
   (c) economic, social and territorial cohesion;
   (d) agriculture and fisheries, excluding the conservation of marine biological resources;
   (e) environment;
   (f) consumer protection;
   (g) transport;
   (h) trans-European networks;
   (i) energy;

   (j) area of freedom, security and justice;
   (k) **common safety concerns in public health matters, for the aspects defined in this Treaty.**

3. In the areas of research, technological development and space, the Union shall have competence to carry out activities, in particular to define and implement programmes; however, the exercise of that competence shall not result in Member States being prevented from exercising theirs.

4. In the areas of development cooperation and humanitarian aid, the Union shall have competence to carry out activities and conduct a common policy; however, the exercise of that competence shall not result in Member States being prevented from exercising theirs.

Article 6

The Union shall have competence to carry out actions to support, coordinate or supplement the actions of the Member States. The areas of such action shall, at European level, be:

   (a) **protection and improvement of human health;**
   (b) industry;
   (c) culture;
   (d) tourism;
   (e) education, vocational training, youth and sport;
   (f) civil protection;
   (g) administrative cooperation.

The powers of the European Commission with respect to public health and consumer protection were increased in the 1990s as part of the negotiations for the Amsterdam Treaty. However, Article 152 about public health explicitly excluded Commission competence with respect to health services. Increasing the EU's role in public health had become less controversial for Member States because of the salmonella and BSE (so-called mad cow disease) public health crises. Furthermore, Member States and public health groups concerned with health promotion saw scope for extending the reach of public health and limiting tobacco advertising under the auspices of the EU. In this respect, further European action for health protection and promotion was not a problem.

The wake-up call for Member States as regards health services came in the form of judgements on health services and internal markets in the context of the European Court of Justice. While these were not new, and could have been anticipated after an early decision on abortion services in the 1980s, the broader implications of these decisions were not necessarily taken in or understood by Member States at that time. However, after the cases of Kohl (ECJ 1998b), Decker (ECJ 1998a) and Watts (ECJ 2006), the consideration of health services as services in the context of internal markets became clear to all types of health system. As views of the European Court of Justice opened scope for policies and expansion for EU competence in services as services within internal markets, the Member States were faced with uncomfortable prospects.

The emergence of these European Court of Justice decisions did not take place in a vacuum, but represented a choice of the Court of Justice to con- sider the rights of individuals over and above those of societies. The decision of the European Court of Justice to focus on constitutional freedoms has strengthened constitutional asymmetry between obligations to free mobility and economic rights on one hand, and social rights and security on the other (Hatzopoulos 2002; Nedwick 2006). Mossialos and colleagues have also noted that the jurisprudence of the European Court of Justice has played a pivotal role in EU-level law- and policy-making in the main areas of Europeanisation, where national welfare systems have been restricted. These include economic and monetary policy, internal market policies, EU employ- ment law, EU law on the free movement of human beings, and health-related regulation (Mossialos et al. 2009).

While the increasing role of the EU in health systems governance should not, in principle, automatically imply the increasing commercialisation of health services, the provisions of the treaties, as well as the interpretation of their implications, have been conducive to this. Furthermore, while governments do liberalise and commercialise health services as result of their own political priorities, EU involvement seems to strengthen and enhance these processes.

Where does the agenda come from?

How health services have become part of the EU policy-making with no explicit treaty basis – and even an explicit treaty basis for exclusion of these from Commission competence – does require an explanation. How was this possible, and why has it taken place? Is it simply a result of spillover from the European legal integration process? For example, Scott Greer has used Haas to explain how European health systems have changed as an example of neofunctionalism (Greer 2006). Neofunctionalism has been seen as the first 'theory' of regional integration. But it has also been rejected or considered obsolescent (Haas 1975; Schmitter 2003), although often remaining part of the frameworks in which analysis is made. What is relevant for health care is that this neofunctionalist type of argumentation would, for example, claim that due to increasing economic interdependence, the establishment of new institutional structures and capacities, and supranational regulatory mea- sures, integration would extend into other areas. Mossialos and colleagues, on the other hand, suggest that part of the challenge is to reconceptualise the relationship of social security/welfare *vis à vis* the internal market, so as to develop robust and helpful contributions from the EU law and policy to health systems governance in Europe (Mossialos et al. 2009).

There was no explicit and outspoken lobbying or support for health services markets from health providers in the 1990s. There was more willingness from some Member States than others to seek EU engagement with health care, but it did not seem to be a major health policy concern. In many countries, decentralised provision of services has resulted in challenges for governance, and EU engagement has been seen as a potential source for additional financing or, where costs were to be controlled, for governance. Although Member States were not particularly eager to increase the European Commission's role in health care, nevertheless it is possible to distinguish five different sets of interests leading in this direction.

1. European Commission and Ministry of Finance interests in controlling health care finance

This was often based on the assumption that more market-driven provision of health care and health care reforms would lower health care costs (see point 4 below), but is also likely to have been influenced by ideas concerning the assumed virtues of small government and the benefits of free markets in general. Social and health care costs have been a concern in European budgetary review processes (European Council 2004). The 2010 report on public finances in the EMU unsurprisingly considers that 'Fiscal consolidation and long-term financial sustainability will need to go hand in hand with important structural reforms, in particular of pension, health care, social protection and education systems' (European Commission 2010a: 5). Health care funding priorities in the context of structural reforms are also discussed under the rubric of the 'modernisation' of health care (Hervey 2008).

2. Broader free-market lobbying forces and interests operating at EU level

These include, for example, the pharmaceutical industry, which often provides support to more market- and industry-oriented health care reforms. While health care-provision industries were neither sufficiently established nor yet very active in the early 1990s, a more commercialised context of health care provision has been emerging and is often supported by other health care-related interest and lobbying groups.[1] Pharmaceutical companies, such as Pfizer, have also been involved in European health care debates (e.g. Luxembourg Ministry of Health et al. 2007). The pharmaceutical company Merck funds the European policy journal *Eurohealth*. Janssen has funded analysis by the Economist Intelligence Unit on the future of European health care (Economist Intelligence Unit 2011). The free market-oriented Stockholm Network has a specific programme for Central and Eastern European (CEE) countries and health care (Stockholm Network 2011). Other European policy actors and think tanks, which favour free market approaches, often have ties to health care-related industry funding, related interest associations, or national or European agencies responsible for competitiveness, industry, trade or investments. Commercialisation-oriented influence on health care policy is often channelled through these more powerful sectoral ministries, and their policies and policy priorities derive from this, rather than being the result of policy priorities within Ministries of Health. This has been evident, for example, in policy changes that have taken place in Finland and Sweden (Tritter et al. 2009), while in the case of England, commercialisation has been more prominently on the agenda of the Department of Health.

3. Institutional interests of DG Sanco and DG Employment in establishing their role and increasing their relevance within the European Commission

Public health action and regulation does not have great prestige or financial clout, but can gain powerful enemies in the tobacco, alcohol, food and advertising industries, because health-related regulatory measures often interfere with their interests and markets. Rather than tinkering with less appealing public health or health-promotion matters, the focus on health services, health technologies and medicines enables a role that fits better with broader Commission interests and strategies, and involves more financial and commercial policy-related issues. As higher-level civil servants in the Commission often serve for a limited time and circulate from one directorate to another, keeping on good terms with the more powerful directorates and actors can be a good career move.

It is thus not surprising that the Commission might define its role more as conveying to Member States the obligations that arise from the Treaties and European strategies for the modernisation of health systems, rather than positioning itself as an actor whose obligations arise from health or health policy concerns. This becomes evident, for example, in the short statement concerning the purpose of the open method of coordination:

> Responsibility for the organisation and funding of the health care and elderly care sector rests primarily with the Member States, **which are bound, when exercising this responsibility, to respect the freedoms defined and the rules laid down in the Treaty**. The added value of the 'open method of coordination' is therefore in the identification of challenges common to all and in support for the Member States' reforms.
>
> (European Commission 2004: 11)

While the open method of coordination (OMC) might be perceived by the Commission as a means for adjusting Member States' health systems to the requirements of rules laid down in the Treaty, there is no strong evidence that OMCs would have pushed towards the liberalisation of health services in practice (Hervey 2008). However, this is unlikely to have been a prominent focus of activities at the outset, since Member States were reluctant to embrace internal market regulations in the area, and because there was a concern over the increasing role of European Commission (see below). However, if the OMC was considered initially as a means for legitimating the EU's role in health care, it did successfully contribute to the recognition of health care as part of EU activities and competence in the context of the Lisbon Treaty negotiations.

4. Assumptions regarding the benefits of market mechanisms and new public management approaches for the public sector

The policy literature and work on public sector reforms and cost management within the public sector are often based on general assumptions regarding the benefits of market mechanisms and new public management approaches for the public sector in general. This way of thinking is also implicit within the European Commission's understanding of, and emphasis on, the 'modernisation' of health care. While the EU may have been a source of influence on these efforts on national-level agendas, it is not necessarily the main or the only one. A broader influence on health care reforms and public management practices is exercised in the context of the Organisation for Economic Co-operation and Development (OECD). This stresses contractual and competitive relationships in public service provision as a means of curbing costs and improving efficiency during the 1980s and 1990s. Such thinking is also inherent in the assumption that Europe-wide health care markets will deliver improved efficiencies through choice. The EU has also actively taken up and promoted a regulatory reform agenda, including 'better' regulation and 'smart' regulation (European Commission 2005, 2010b), which strengthens the role of business interests and competitiveness considerations and, more or less explicitly, supports deregulation.

5. Constitutionalisation of European treaties and the importance given to the European Court of Justice

The final interest is seen in the process of constitutionalisation of European treaties, and the importance given to the European Court of Justice and treaties for establishing legitimacy and the framework for change as a technical and neutral matter, in comparison with active, explicit and more contestable actions in the context of political programmes and cooperation. In this respect, the Maastricht Treaty and later the Lisbon Treaty have been important in defining and framing the context of EU action and, in particular, the respective competences between Member States on the one hand and the Commission on the other. How competence is defined and interpreted is important for the Commission, since it sets the context in which it has to operate. Subsidiarity[2] is still emphasised and recognised in the European context, but constitutional change in terms of how and by whom shared competence is defined – and therefore how subsidiarity is also defined – is likely to be of more importance, even though this may not have been properly understood by Member States during negotiation of the Lisbon Treaty.

European Commission and Member States

The commercialisation of health systems was thus not – at least openly – a particular agenda for anyone. However, it can be said that at the end of 1990s, three policy 'streams' supporting commercialisation directly or indirectly did merge in terms that fit Kingdon's idea of policy streams (Kingdon 1984). These are first, the need to curb the public costs of health systems due to the increasing needs of ageing societies; second, the increasing perception in public policy management circles of markets and competition as a mechanism of change and a way of improving efficiency; and third, the interest of the European Commission in engaging in health services oversight and regulation. While structural funds can be used for health, the responsibility of Member States to finance health systems has not been directly addressed or challenged. From the Commission's point of view, it is likely to have been more important to be able to regulate how and under what terms health care systems are financed, organised and regulated at national level.

Member States have not been very interested in further engagement with the EU over the governance of health services, but it is likely that some of them have seen the mediation of Europe-level regulatory powers as a way of gaining oversight of decentralised services. The legitimacy of the increasing role of the European Commission in health was, to a large extent, 'sold' to Member States, first as the lesser of two evils and an alternative to having 'the European Court of Justice in the driver's seat', and second as a response to the increasing mobility of Europeans with holiday homes and residences in other Member States, prompting a focus on cross-border care. Patient cross-border mobility has also enabled the Commission to engage with patients' associations and to frame European policies as being in the interest of patients and patients' rights (for example in the Directive on Patients' Rights; see below).

The mobility of Europeans has been accommodated on the basis of the regulation on coordination of social security systems (Regulation 1971: 2; 2004). However, the increasing mobility of the elderly within Europe, for example to Spain, has underlined the need to understand the nature of the problem as well as the extent to which the financing burden needs to be shared. Thus it is not surprising that the first moves in the area of patient mobility were initiated during the Spanish presidency in 2002.

The decisions of the European Court of Justice became the legitimation for the initial inclusion of health services as part of the Services Directive, situating health services rather squarely as part of the internal markets, under provisions governing internal markets. Health services were treated just like any other services. While Member States and European Parliament members carved out health services from the Services Directive, at the same time they gave further legitimacy and rights to DG Sanco to engage with the Health Services Directive. This was at the time perceived as the lesser evil in comparison with the European Court of Justice or DG Internal Markets. It is unlikely that when they did this, Member States anticipated that it would be brought back under internal market articles. Furthermore, as discussed below, the Council's conclusions on common values and health systems explicitly articulated opposition to this.

The emphasis on the ageing population and the consequences for financing was given as a further reason for introducing an OMC to address this matter. It is not accidental that the first OMC was on long-term care, since an OMC that addressed health care directly would have been unlikely to succeed. As a process, the open method of coordination is a relatively weak and soft power mechanism, but it is an established way of acting, and can be used to initiate administrative cooperation or otherwise pave the way to gaining acceptability for the changes and reforms that are sought. It can also be viewed as a process whereby Member State administrations can be introduced to each other in order to further European cooperation in the area. It is not accidental that health services were first mentioned in this context in the Lisbon Treaty.

During the Lisbon Treaty negotiations, Member States had the option of changing the Treaty so as to create an exception for health services, but this did not happen. While some Member States, including Finland, Sweden and the UK, did engage with efforts in the area, it was not part of the 'high politics' agenda of the negotiations, and was thought not to merit a strong negotiation stand. It is probable that a lack of understanding, or the low importance accorded to the implications of what was being negotiated, led to the situation where the Lisbon Treaty encouraged further Commission action in this area. For example, the UK Foreign and Commonwealth Office's analysis of the Treaty of Lisbon in comparison with prior treaties states that new public health article 168:

> Draws on Article 152 TEC. Extends the scope and focus of the EU activities, but includes a stronger reference to Member States' responsibility for definition of their health policies and management of health services.
> (Foreign and Commonwealth Office 2008: 14)

The fact that the Commission chose to proceed further with some of the substantive issues it could not accommodate in Article 168 implies that this was a matter of key interest. Furthermore, the extension of competence to health services went ahead, despite the fact that it could be argued to be contrary to the principles of subsidiarity and proportionality. The regulation on coordination of social security often provides better access to care for residents in other countries than the new Directive on Patients' Rights. The financial costs of cross-border care, acknowledged by the Commission, have been estimated to be of the magnitude of 1 percent of total health care costs (European Commission 2008a). The establishment of the new Directive on Patients' Rights under internal markets provisions gave the Commission scope to prioritise its areas of interest utilising the newly defined shared competence after the Lisbon Treaty.

The Commission has thus taken an active stance on health services, where policies have made more progress than in public health and health promotion, even though action in public health is considered more favourably by Member States, if not actively promoted by them (Koivusalo 2010). For example, although ensuring a high level of health protection in all policies is a Treaty commitment under Article 168, this has received relatively little attention and has not been at the core of the more deregulatory emphasis on 'better' and 'smart' regulation.

Member States and health proponents wake up – but only briefly

The carving out of health services from the Services Directive was an important reminder of the limits and willingness of Member States to take health services to the internal markets. Furthermore, to make this explicit Member States issued a statement on common values.

> This is a statement by the 25 Health Ministers of the European Union, about the common values and principles that underpin Europe's health systems. We believe such a statement is important in providing clarity for our citizens, and timely, because of the recent vote of the Parliament and the revised proposal of the Commission to remove healthcare from the proposed Directive on Services in the Internal Market. We strongly believe that developments in this area should result from political consensus, and not solely from case law.
>
> We also believe that it will be important to safeguard the common values and principles outlined below as regards the application of competition rules on the systems that implement them.
>
> (European Council 2006: 146/2)

The emphasis on management of health systems with respect to national and EU-level governance also made clear that:

> This statement sets out the common values and principles that are shared across the European Union about how health systems respond to the needs of the populations and patients that they serve. It also explains that the practical ways in which these values and principles become a reality in the health systems of the EU vary significantly between Member States, and will continue to do so. **In particular, decisions about the basket of healthcare to which citizens are entitled and the mechanisms used to finance and deliver that healthcare, such as the**

**extent to which it is appropriate to rely on market mechanisms and
competitive pressures to manage health systems must be taken in the
national context.**

(European Council 2006: 2)

However, hopes with respect to the values and priorities of health systems were
short-lived as the Commission leaked a proposal for effective cross-border
services. Due to the controversial approach of a number of provisions in the
leaked version, including reference to Article 95 on the functioning of internal markets as the basis for its legitimacy, the proposed directive remained
shelved for a year. It was eventually released alongside other more social pro-
tection-oriented documents in July 2008. In the meantime, the name had
been changed from one that emphasised effective cross-border care to one
that centred on patients' rights.

The proposed directive made reference to Council conclusions on common
values, but neither these nor patient rights were reflected in the actual
content of the Commission communication. At the end of the day, the
communication was concerned more with establishing health care markets
through enabling choice in health care, as well as limiting the scope of
Member States to require pre-authorisation before citizens could seek care
in another Member State. In establishing common standards for what a
patient can expect to be reimbursed for, it also opened up the possibility of
exit from national health care systems. The Commission proposal for the
directive redefines and establishes common principles as part of the directive,
and assigns to Member States the task of harmonizing and legitimating action:

> As recognised by the Member States in the Council Conclusions on
> Common values and principles in European Union Health Systems
> there is a set of operating principles that are shared by health systems
> throughout the Community ... /. ... It is therefore appropriate to
> require that it is the authorities of the Member State on whose territory
> the healthcare is provided, who are responsible for ensuring compliance
> with those operating principles. This is necessary to ensure the con-
> fidence of patients in cross-border healthcare, which is itself necessary for
> achieving patients' mobility and free movement of provision of healthcare
> in the internal market as well as a high level of health protection.
>
> (European Commission 2008: 23)

There is no doubt that the market-making aspects of the proposed directive,
as well as the fact that it used the legal basis of the internal market Article 95
as the basis for its own legitimacy, contradicted the aims and focus of
Council conclusions on common values. The directive was also a concern
for several Member States, to the extent that until late 2010, the proposed
directive was stuck in the Council of the European Union. Even when it was
passed in the Council, the Austrian, Polish, Portuguese and Romanian

delegations voted against it, while the Slovak delegation abstained (European Council 2011a).

The reasons for Member States' disagreement included the potential financial and legal consequences of the directive, which in practice enables patients to seek care from the private sector in another country and still be reimbursed from public funds. The financial consequences of the required changes are expected to be more manageable in a social insurance or private insurance system, whereas for locally established NHS-type services this is a potential problem on two grounds. First, if the numbers of those who exit increase, it will end up taking resources out of the system, while services still need to be maintained. Second, it creates a bargaining ground for national private-sector providers for eligibility for reimbursement. For example, where responsibilities for financing are defined on the basis of people living in a given area, the movement of patients to another country or area is likely to take resources out of the pool intended to reimburse services for that given population. At the same time, compensating savings cannot be made, as health centres and hospitals cannot be closed in order to maintain services for the rest of the population. A concrete example is Italy, where fiscal decentralisation has led to concerns over the equity implications of patient mobility (Ferrario and Zanardi 2009; Senese 2008). Even if the cost implications of mobility of patients are small, establishing rights to use private services in another country puts pressure on extending choice within local services and the reimbursement of use of private services at local level as well. This is because it is likely to be untenable in the long term to reimburse the use of private services outside, but not within, a country. Analyses of Member States actions so far suggest that they have tried to cope with the marginal changes in the area so as to avoid Commission infringement, but without encouraging cross-border care (Baeten et al. 2010)

The aim of market-making was inherent in many provisions of the proposed directive and, in particular, in the early leaked versions of the proposal. One key provision has dealt with the extent to which Member States can require prior authorisation for seeking care from another country. For example, Member States wanted to maintain the right to require that patients seek prior authorisation for hospital or other high-cost care if they go abroad. This had already been a concern during discussions on the Services Directive, as it would have affected the capacity of Member States to plan and govern national health systems.

The importance of market-making and the removal of limits to pre-authorisation is reflected in the fact that the Commission itself actively intervened in seeking to limit the scope of Member States to require prior authorisation through initiating a European Court of Justice case against France (ECJ 2008). France had required prior authorisation for use of costly medical technology, although this did not require a hospital stay. The European Commission considered this to represent a breach of free movement. However, by this time the European Court of Justice was a source of support to the Member States against Commission complaints. Against Commission claims, the European Court of Justice ruled in favour of allowing the retention of capacities to plan and anticipate costs through pre-authorisation as a condition for reimbursement of very expensive costs in another Member State, even if provision of these services did not always take place in a hospital.

Politics matter

European policies or EU policies involve not simply the politics of Member States against European institutions, but politics that are formed and governed in the context of particular regimes and national priorities. A case in point is Sweden, which, under the social democratic reign, had a highly critical attitude to internal markets and health services. Together with the UK Labour government and the Social Democratic Party-led coalition government in Finland, it sought to limit the EU powers in the area of health services and commercial policy during the Lisbon Treaty negotiations. On the other hand, the centre-right conservative-led government in Sweden has been more embracing of health systems and internal markets and trade, with a more permissive – if not actively promoting – approach to the role of the EU and its actions, for example in the context of the proposed Directive on Patients' Rights.

The emphasis on the liberalisation of services and a more free-market approach tends to be supported more frequently by traditionally right-wing policy actors. The market-making and shaping influence of the EU may seem technical or judicially driven, but it is not without its political underpinnings. On the contrary, it can be said that the constitutionalisation of supranational legal governance with respect to a commercial, policy-driven agenda and a constitution that is tilted in favour of liberalisation is a deeply political matter. On the other hand, the shift of health politics and regulation to the European level has also been seen as one aspect of governments coping with governance in a context of increasing decentralisation. In terms of national decision-making, European policy-making enables a shift of responsibilities and regulatory burden in the direction of the EU on one hand, and of costs and obligations to the local level and to individuals on the other.

The implicit approach to health care in the EU often emphasises the residual role of public services. These are tacitly considered as services of little or no commercial interest, whereas all other services are to be part of internal markets. The extent to which European policies, and the rather residual social policy focus of these policies, have managed to maintain the support of left-leaning and social democratic governments is striking. This has remained despite the free-market and private-sector interest-promoting internal market agenda and innovation policies, and the public policy impacts of public spending control and cuts, which have been required by EMU policies. The critique of the EU has been left in the hands of either those who consider the EU to be 'too social', and who would prefer even more market-oriented policies (e.g. UKIP in the UK), or those who otherwise are more value conservative, espousing nationalistic and populistic policies. The liberal economic agenda at the EU level has thus not been questioned to the extent that policy contents promoted at European level might imply, when viewed from a welfare state and health policy perspective.

Furthermore, economic and financial crisis and problems with the euro have – so far – strengthened rather than weakened economic integration, and have further tightened public finances, with a stronger focus on economic competitiveness, growth and innovation, which also has relevance for health policy development in the EU.

European health policies as a means of innovation and economic growth

The establishment of European competence in the field of health care has taken place through incremental policy changes, often legitimated on the basis of concern over health care costs. The mobility of patients is not the only aspect of health systems that has become part of European policy, but should be considered as a starting point. The EU has already drawn up a green paper on the European workforce and health, which is likely to be of importance in future (European Commission 2008b). The European Commission is also likely to engage more extensively with policies that affect the regulation and financing of health services as part of policy developments in the areas of government procurement, internal market functioning, and principles of freedom of establishment and freedom to provide cross-border services,[3] and as part of emerging engagement with investment policies (European Commission 2010b). The European Commission has also launched a communication on the EU's role in global health (European Commission 2010c).

The issue of free mobility in the EU has also brought to many Member States the realisation that this may affect capacities to retain and regulate the workforce, and to regulate and control the costs of care. While health care markets have been envisaged as a potential commercial sector for the newer Member States, they may in practice be facing greater pressure from the mobility of the health workforce (discussed below). Another aspect has been the challenges faced when governments have sought to reverse from privatisation policies. Poland and Slovakia have both been challenged by commitments to investment treaties as they have sought to withdraw from privatisation programmes (Hall 2010). The European Commission has also been interested in whether Slovakian measures have contravened the EU principle of free movement of capital (Hall 2010).

However, in contrast to the needs and concerns of Member States in controlling health care costs and maintaining budgetary oversight, health care systems are increasingly coming to be seen as a means of supporting policies that seek to promote innovation and economic growth. In this context, health systems are no longer considered as public services, but often more importantly as a basis for commercial growth. While aspects of this type of thinking have been on the European agenda since the original emphasis on 'health is wealth' during the reflection process (Byrne 2004), it has found new forms in Commission activities. It has also been reiterated in the context of the new emphasis on 'health for growth'.

The preparatory work for the pilot project on active and healthy ageing was carried out – not in DG Sanco – but in the context of competitiveness with related Member State Council conclusions for the pilot project, published in March 2011 (European Council 2011b). One of the explicit aims of the European Innovation Partnership is to foster competitiveness and the growth of businesses (European Commission 2011). Related input on the sustainable financing of health systems appeared on the Council agenda of EU Member States in May 2011, with an emphasis on 'modern, responsive and sustainable health systems'. The initial wording clearly saw health care as a 'driver and contributor to growth', and pointed to a need for new models of health care to overcome existing challenges, and for establishment of a reflection group drawn from other sectors in order to guide this process. While the final conclusions are a watered-down version of the original text (European Council 2011c), establishing the reflection process is likely to lead to further suggestions as to how health care can serve the needs of economic growth and contribute to the 2020 strategy. The first indications from the budgetary document suggest that the Commission is to fund a new 'health for growth' programme, which will be 'oriented towards actions with clear EU added value, in line with the Europe 2020 objectives and new legal obligations' (European Commission 2011a, 2011b).

While the good news might be that investments in health are recognised in the context of economic policies and competitiveness, the bad news is that this may not imply increasing public funding, as health systems are more likely to be considered as a means and ground for enhancing entrepreneurialism and competitiveness.

There is nothing to imply that DG Sanco would not continue to consider as its task conveying EU policy priorities to Member States and ensuring they do not engage in measures that could be against Commission commitments on other, higher priorities. The ability to use structural funds for health gives some capacity to the European Commission for supporting and initiating projects that it considers important. However, it might be time to reflect on what kind of political and policy changes the European Commission's current interests in health suggest these are likely to be.

In a multi-level governance, where costs are paid predominantly by Member States, there is a danger that more general lobbying groups keen on promoting the free market, as well as views from pharmaceutical and e-health industries, which are interested in securing financing of investments, will gain priority more easily in the work of the European Commission, over and above health policy considerations or the scope for sustainable health care financing. While responsibilities for health systems financing might still remain with Member States, the issue of how, and on what basis, this takes place requires further attention.

The paradox is that, despite Member States' interests in controlling costs, measures taken at EU level are likely to increase the very costs these measures were initially introduced to control. This implies that cost-sharing by users is likely to increase rather than decrease within European health care systems in the future. This would be in line with the emphasis on market-making and on consumer choice and mobility within European markets.

There is also an increasing number of lobbyists working at the EU level with free-market or commercial policy goals. The role of international networks and think tanks is interesting. For example, one active participant in health policy debates at the EU level is Health Consumer Powerhouse, whose founder and president, Johan Hjertqvist, has a background of a trade association for private health care organisations and heading the health policy unit at Timbro, a Swedish think tank with offices in Stockholm and Brussels (Hjertqvist 2003, 2008). Despite its name, Health Consumer Powerhouse, which makes comparisons across European Member States on the basis of pre-set criteria, and does not disclose information on funding, is likely to be funded by the pharmaceutical industry or other corporate interest organisations. Health Consumer Powerhouse has been actively and openly promoting health care markets in Europe and on the European Commission agenda. This emphasis was reflected in a *Wall Street Journal* interview with Mr Hjertqvist, which states that: 'People are gradually realizing monopoly-style systems are becoming obsolete and unaffordable, Mr. Hjertqvist says. Health care should be looked at as the largest industry in Europe but instead it has for too long been regarded as an administrative operation' (Espinoza 2011).

As public resources are limited, the reality is that there is potential for expanding spending on health compared with, for example, the United States, as Europeans still spend a smaller share of GDP on health than the United States. It is likely that people are more willing to accept paying more for health and health security in comparison with other consumer goods or services. For those seeking commercial opportunities, there is scope for influencing government spending on health so that it is done in ways that support private sector and commercial entrepreneurs as part of the pursuit for competitiveness and growth.

The role and relevance of CEE countries in the process

The scope for using structural funds in support of health systems could be important for CEE countries, which are likely to face high costs of health technologies and care, an ageing population, and health workforce scarcity. On the other hand, the focus and the use of structural funds for the 'modernisation' of health care or for health-related investments could suggest that this could also form a basis for a variety of clientele, including all those who market services and products for health administration. The ways in which structural funds are used, and the results, depend on priorities and decisions at national level. While structural funds can become resources to finance primarily commercial operators,[4] these may also be used to enhance other functions, such as diminishing inequalities in health.

CEE countries have a background of health care reforms prior to accession, with the involvement of the World Bank and bilateral and international donors. In terms of the privatisation of health care or changing of health systems, the role of the EU has been of limited significance:

> The policy design recommendations were often based on the specific experience and knowledge of the international experts in their own countries or elsewhere in the world. The major players in the CEE/CIS healthcare reforms have been the World Bank, followed by USAID, WHO, and to lesser extent by Western European governments. Thus, the American influence via the WB and US government-funded programs has been predominant in the region.
>
> (Shakarishvili and Davey 2005: 15).

This is compatible with views in relation to pension reforms. For example, Orenstein has pointed out how the EU influence on pension reforms in CEE countries was limited, if not entirely absent, in comparison with global campaigning and the role of the World Bank (Orenstein 2008). On the other hand, a more progressive emphasis on ensuring universal access has been associated with joining the EU, and in particular with the role of European Charter on Social Rights. The response to more market-oriented health care reforms before accession to the EU is reflected in the 1996 Ljubljana Charter, which takes a strong stand against such efforts. The Ljubljana Charter was, however, not signed by the UK or the Czech Republic. However, analysis of politics of the Czech Republic and health care reforms also makes evident the role of national politics and policy-makers. For example, the Czech Republic declined funding in spite of undertaking major reforms and priva-tisation measures (Ovseiko 2008). While recognising the role of national politics in the process, the politics of reform would support views as to the broader influence of external actors on national policy choices and options in the region (see e.g. Deacon and Hulse 1997; Wedel 1998).

The role of private sector foundations, think tanks, networks and policy operators is also important in the context of the EU politics. While earlier experimentation since the early 1990s on more market-oriented approaches led to the Ljubljana Charter, which was critical of solely market-driven approaches (Ljubljana Charter 1996), there is an emerging interest amongst think tanks in the area. The programme of the Stockholm Network CEEAHEAD, for example, suggests responding to financial crisis pressures by devising 'new ways of providing health care', notably:

> By encouraging open competition in healthcare, CEE governments will be able to develop a healthcare environment that is more receptive to

patients and which obligates providers and insurers to offer high-quality services that will look favourable in comparison to other alternatives;

By allowing greater use of public–private partnerships, CEE governments could bring about an improvement in the quality of healthcare services, whilst lowering the cost burden on the public purse. Furthermore, by opening health care systems up to more private initiative, patients in the CEE region could benefit from a healthcare system that is designed around their needs and choices;

By fostering more varied sources of healthcare funding through allowing private health insurance to work more closely alongside social insurance, CEE governments could bring about greater patient choice and empowerment. In doing so, patients in the CEE region would be given the power to choose a healthcare plan that suits their needs and circumstances, whilst maintaining a public safety net for those unable to contribute.

(Healy et al. 2010: 8)

While presented in the form of patient empowerment and choice, the proposals effectively seek to break with any existing mechanisms for cross-subsidisation within health systems. While presented as a solution to financial crisis and service to patients, it is clear that what is suggested is further commercialisation in ways that are not known to reduce costs of care. The emphasis on choice and patient empowerment fits with similar discourse in the UK, Sweden and Finland (Tritter et al. 2009), but is in stark contrast with measures known to save money.

The process of privatisation is, however, clearly in the interest of health care market operators within Europe, while privatisation policies have struggled with popular opposition to the privatisation of hospitals. This is reflected, for example, in market analysts' views on future options for private health care markets:

As these countries transitioned from centrally organised to decentralised healthcare systems, there has been significant resistance to private health-care; many citizens consider healthcare a service that should be provisioned 'free of charge' by the state. This is exemplified by the ongoing discussion on privatisation of hospitals in Poland or the deep dissatisfaction of Czechs once the mandatory fees for publicly provisioned services were introduced in 2008.

Market participants need to provide objective information and educational campaigns about healthcare privatisation to convince societies about the benefits of private healthcare. Companies able to effectively address the gaps that have not been fulfilled by the public healthcare system are positioned to make strong revenue gains.

(Grzywinska 2010: 1).

On the other hand, the free mobility of the European workforce and patients is no longer assumed to benefit all Member States, or the new Member States in particular. Retaining a workforce on lower salaries is likely to become an increasing challenge alongside the potential entrepreneurial possibilities that health services can provide in the private sector. The financial crisis and related austerity measures have also resulted in reports of increasing numbers of medical doctors heading west. Growing numbers of physicians, surgeons, anaesthesists and other specialists from Bulgaria, Hungary and Romania are said to be packing up for countries such as the UK, Germany and Sweden (Molnar 2011).

The changing context of health policy surfaced during the Hungarian presidency, when a special meeting addressed the problem in Gödöllö on 6 April 2011. In particular, the Gödöllö meeting raised the Hungarian government's concerns over retaining their workforce. The discussion also indicated that for medical professionals, salary differences could be sixfold. It is already anticipated that the migration of health personnel will affect CEE countries more severely than elsewhere. For example, migration intentions in Estonia have been high for a long time, and in the early 2000s these were also accompanied by active recruitment on the part of Scandinavian countries (Vörk et al. 2004).

However, calls for the European Commission to help retain health professionals within countries might be a misplaced hope on the part of Ministries of Health. Retaining the health workforce runs counter to EU Treaty provisions with respect to free mobility. On the other hand, if health workforce scarcity becomes a political matter, the European Commission might gain an interest in solving the problem on the basis of importing workforces from poorer countries outside the EU. Such workforces are readier to trade professional services for lower salaries. The EU is, for example, negotiating a bilateral free trade agreement with India, which, together with a number of other Asian countries, has an active interest in exporting healthcare workers.

While new Member States may have earlier been supportive of more market-led developments, the difficulties for CEE countries posed by free mobility and the commercialisation of health care are also becoming clearer. The new Member States are likely to face the challenge of either going with the market, and seeking to benefit as much as possible from the EU support on the way, or alternatively moving more in the direction of national policy priorities, which may or may not support a less commercialised health care system.

Towards European health care markets?

The current focus of EU activity is likely to push European health care policies towards further commercialisation, and potentially towards a situation comparable to that in the United States. While health systems evolve on the basis of the national historical and political context, the role of the EU is likely to be important, especially for smaller and poorer Member States.

The context of multi-level governance is a challenge for policies pursued within the EU. While commitments with respect to social rights and the social charter may push the focus towards the universal provision of services, the stronger constitutional emphasis on freedom of movement, and the prominence of internal market and competitiveness priorities within the European Commission, are likely to further enhance the commercialisation of health care.

While an argument can be made for the relevance of health systems to economic growth, there is a danger that, in the current European context, health systems will increasingly be treated as a site for the development of commercial interests and economic growth.

European citizens and Member States have common concerns over the values and principles on the basis of which their health systems function. The issue is not so much that there are different priorities in Ministries of Health in different Member States as it is a question of the politics of European integration and how this is shaped within countries. It is thus about not only the distribution of power and competence between the EU and Member States, but what European policies imply for public policies and interests on the one hand, and health-related corporate policy and policy interests on the other.

Notes

1 Our follow-up and interviews with European actors would support these views. It is likely, also, as the number of actors with interests in health care provision markets was limited or they were only emerging onto the European policy scene. However, this is likely to be a growing market, already with large-scale actors such as Capio, as well as other emerging corporate actors with interests in the area.

2 The European Union's online glossary defines subsidiarity as follows: 'The principle of subsidiarity is defined in Article 5 of the Treaty on European Union. It ensures that decisions are taken as closely as possible to the citizen and that constant checks are made to verify that action at Union level is justified in light of the possibilities available at national, regional or local level. Specifically, it is the principle whereby the Union does not take action (except in the areas that fall within its exclusive competence), unless it is more effective than action taken at national, regional or local level. It is closely bound up with the principle of proportionality, which requires that any action by the Union should not go beyond what is necessary to achieve the objectives of the Treaties.' (http://europa.eu/legislation_summaries/glossary/subsidiarity_en.htm)

3 On freedom of establishment (Article 49) and the freedom to provide cross-border services (Article 56), see e.g. http://ec.europa.eu/internal_market/services/principles_en.htm

4 European Union funds, including structural and cohesion funds, can be used to support the local private sector or to provide infrastructure or support policies. For example, the European Federation of Pharmaceutical Industries and Associations (EFPIA) already gives guidance on the matter (www.efpia.eu/Content/Default.asp?PageID=559&DocID=5677).

References

Baeten, R., Vanhercke, B. and Coucheir, M. (2010) *The Europeanisation of National Health Care Systems: Creative Adaptation in the Shadow of Patient Mobility Case Law*, OSE Paper No. 3, Brussels: European Social Observatory.

Byrne, D. (2004) 'Enabling good health for all. A reflection process for a new EU health strategy', Brussels: European Commission. http://ec.europa.eu/health/phoverview/Documents/byrnereflectionen.pdf

Deacon, B. and Hulse, M. (1997) 'The making of post-communist social policy: the role of international agencies', *Journal of Social Policy*, 26: 43–62.

Economist Intelligence Unit (2011) 'The future of healthcare in Europe'. www.businessresearch.eiu.com/future-healthcare-europe.html-0

Espinoza, J. (2011) 'Europe's failing health', *Wall Street Journal*, March 28. http://online.wsj.com/article/SB10001424052748704893604576200724221948728.html?KEYWORDS=javier+espinoza

European Commission (2004) *Modernising Social Protection for the Development of High Quality, Accessible and Sustainable Health Care and Long-term Care: Support for the National Strategies Using 'The Open Method of Coordination'*, Brussels: European Commission, April 20, COM (2004) final.

——(2005) *Better Regulation for Growth and Jobs in European Union*, Brussels: European Commission, March 16, COM (2005) 97 final.

——(2008a) *Proposal for the Directive on the Application of Patient Rights in Cross-Border Care*, Brussels: European Commission, July 2, COM(2008) 414 final.http://ec.europa.eu/health/ph_overview/co_operation/healthcare/docs/COM_en.pdf

——(2008b) *Green Paper on the European Workforce on Health*, *Brussels: European Commission*, Brussels: European Commission, December 10, COM(2008) 725 final.

——(2010a) *Public Finances in EMU 2010*, Brussels: European Commission. http://ec.europa.eu/economyfinance/pulications/europeaneconomy/2010/pdf/ee-2010-4en.pdf

——(2010b) *Smart Regulation*, Brussels: European Commission, October 8, COM (2010) 543 final.

——(2010c) *Towards a Comprehensive International Investment Policy*, Brussels: European Commission, July 7, COM (2010) 343 final.

——(2010d) *The EU Role In Global Health*, Brussels: European Commission, March 31, COM (2010) 128 final. http://ec.europa.eu/development/icenter/repository/COMM_PDF_COM_2010_0128_EN.PDF

——(2011a) *Public Consultation on the Pilot European Innovation Partnership on Active and Healthy Ageing*, Brussels: European Commission, http://ec.europa.eu/health/ageing/consultations/ageing_cons_01_en.htm

——(2011b) *A Budget for Europe 2020 – Part II: Policy Fiches*, Brussels: European Commission, June 29, COM (2011) 500 final.

——(2011c) *Proposal for a Regulation of the European Parliament and of the Council on Establishing a Health for Growth Programme, the Third Multi-Annual Programme of EU Action in the Field of Health for the Period 2014–20*, Brussels: European Commission, November 9, COM (2011) 709 final.

European Council (2004) *The 2004 Update of the Broad Guidelines of the Economic Policies of the Member States and the Community (for the 2003–5) Period*, Brussels: European Council, June 21, 10676/04.

——(2006) 'Council conclusions on common values and principles in European Union health systems', *Official Journal of the European Union*, C-146/1, June 22. http://eur-lex.europa.eu/LexUriServ/LexUriServ.do?uri=OJ:C:2006:146:0001:0003:EN:PDF

——(2011a) 'Directive on cross-border care adopted', Brussels: Council of the European Union, February 28, 7056/11. www.consilium.europa.eu/uedocs/cms_data/docs/pressdata/en/lsa/119514.pdf

——(2011b) *Conclusions on the Preparatory Work for the Pilot European Innovation Partnership 'Active and Healthy Aging'*, 3074th Competitiveness Council, Brussels: Council of the European Union, March 9.

——(2011c) 'Council conclusions towards modern, responsive and sustainable health systems', *Official Journal of the European Union* C-202/10, July 8.

ECJ (1998a) 'Case C-120/95', Nicolas Decker v. Caisse de Maladie des Employés Privés, European Court of Justice, April 28.

——(1998b) 'Case C-158/96', Raymond Kohll v. Union des Caisses de Maladie, European Court of Justice, April 28.

——(2006) 'Case C-372/04', Yvonne Watts v. Bedford Primary Care Trust, European Court of Justice, May 16.

——(2010) 'Case C-512/08', European Commission v. French Republic, European Court of Justice, October 5.

Ferrario, C. and Zanardi, A. (2009) 'What happens to interregional redistribution as decentralisation goes on?: evidence from the Italian NHS'. www.sie.univpm.it/incontri/rsa50/papers/Ferrario-Zanardi.pdf

Foreign and Commonwealth Office (2008) *A Comparative Table of the Current EC and EU Treaties as Amended by the Treaty of Lisbon*, Norwich: HMSO.

Greer, S. (2006) 'Uninvited Europeanisation: neofunctionalism and the EU in health policy', *Journal of European Public Policy*, 13(1): 134–52.

Grzywinska, D. (2010) 'Private health care markets in CEE countries and Russia to maintain high growth rate through 2016', Frost & Sullivan. www.frost.com/prod/servlet/cpo/223107394.htm

Haas, E.B. (1975) *The Obsolescence of Regional Integration Theory*, Berkeley, CA: Berkeley Press.

Hall, D. (2010) 'Challenges to Slovakia and Poland health policy decisions: use of investment treaties to claim compensation for reversal of privatisation/liberalisation policies', PSIRU, January. www.psiru.org

Hatzopoulos, V. (2002) 'Killing national health and insurance system but *healing* patients? The European market for health care services after the judgements of ECJ in *Vanbraekel and Peerbooms*', *Common Market Law Review*, 39(4): 683–729.

Healy, D., Pugatch, D. and Disney, H. (2010) 'Weathering the storm. Central and Eastern European healthcare in financial crisis', CEE AHEAD, Stockholm Network.

Hervey, T. (2008) 'The European Unions' governance of healthcare and the welfare modernization agenda', *Regulation & Governance*, 2: 103–20.

Hjertqvist, J. (2003) *The End of the Beginning. Health Care Revolution in Stockholm, Part 2*. www.timbro.se/bokhandel/health/pdf/TheEndOfTheBeginning.pdf

Hjertqvist, J. (2008) Johan Hjertqvist, C.V. November 11. www.healthpowerhouse.com/index.php?option=com_content&view=article&id=5&Itemid=

Kingdon, J. W. (1984) *Agendas, Alternatives, and Public Policies*, Boston, MA: Little, Brown

Koivusalo, M. (2010) 'Constitutional issues in European health policy and practice', in K. Tuori and S. Sankari (eds) *The Many Constitutions of Europe*, Farnham: Ashgate.

Ljubljana Charter (1996) *Ljubljana Charter on reforming health care in Europe*, Copenhagen: WHO/Europe. EUR/ICP/CARE9401/CNOI Rev.1. www.euro.who.int/data/assets/pdffile/0010/113302/E55363.pdf

Luxembourg Ministry of Health, Sitra and the Finnish Innovation Fund with Pfizer, Inc. (2007) *Financing Sustainable Health Care in Europe: New Approaches for New Outcomes*. http://elibrary.zdrave.net/document/EU/Commission%20of%20the%20EC/eure324972771_en.pdf

Molnar, G. (2011) 'Frustrated Eastern European doctors head west', AFP/*Google News*, March 31. www.google.com/hostednews/afp/article/ALeqM5gT9q9XQA_nCProjQG_ay6-RAtmPQ?docId=CNG.aecc32d05117083937e1ddc1b7482bef.4e1

Mossialos, E., Permanand, G., Baeten, R. and Hervey, T.K. (eds) *Health Systems Governance in Europe: The Role of European Union Law and Policy*, Cambridge: Cambridge University Press.

Nedwick, C. (2006) 'Citizenship, free movement and health care: cementing individual rights by corroding social solidarity', *Common Market Law Review*, 43(6): 1645–68.

Orenstein, M.A. (2008) 'Out-liberalizing the EU: pension privatization in Central and Eastern Europe', *Journal of European Public Policy*, 15(6): 899–917.

Ovseiko, P.V. (2008) 'The politics of health care reform in central and eastern Europe: the case of the Czech Republic', PhD thesis, Oxford University.

Regulation (1971) Regualtion (EC) 1408/1971 of the Council (on the application of social security schemes to self-employed persons and to members of their families moving within the community), *Official Journal of the European Union*, OJL 149, 5.7.1971.

Regulation (2004) Regualtion (EC) 883/2004 of the European Parliament and the Council (on the coordination of social security systems), *Official Journal of the European Union*, L166/1, 30.4.2004.

Senese, F. (2008) 'Has decentralisation of health care in Italy affected horizontal equity?', poster. www.europubhealth.org/newsletter/news9/poster-francesca-senese.pdf

Schmitter, P.C. (2003) 'Neo-neofunctionalism', in A. Wiener and T. Diez (eds) *European Integration Theory*, Oxford: Oxford University Press.

Shakarishvili, G. and Davey, K. (2008) 'Trends in reforming the provision and financing of healthcare services in CEE/CIS regions during the 1990s', in G. Shakarishvili and K. Davey (eds) *Decentralisation in Health Care*, Budapest: Open Society Institute.

Stockholm Network (2011) CEEAHEAD. www.stockholm-network.org/Conferences-and-Programmes/Health-and-Welfare/CEE-Ahead

Tritter, J.Q., Koivusalo, M., Ollila, E. and Dorfman, P. (2009) *Globalisation, Markets, and Healthcare Policy: Redrawing the Patient as Consumer*, New York: Routledge.

Wedel, J.R. (1998) *Collision and Collusion. The Strange Case of Western Aid to Eastern Europe 1989–1998*, New York: St Martin's Press.

Vörk, A., Kallaste, E. and Priinits, M. (2004) *Migration Intentions of Health Care Professionals: The Case of Estonia*. www.praxis.ee/fileadmin/tarmo/Projektid/Too-ja_Sotsiaal poliitika/Tervishoiutootajate_migratsioon_Eestist/11_labour_Migration.pdf

6 Catastrophic citizenship and discourses of disguise: aspects of health care change in Poland[1]

Peggy Watson

Introduction

Over the past two decades, divisions have taken shape in Poland that have given rise to high levels of social tension. Huge inequalities have been created, and health care changes have brought those inequalities very close to the bone. The raising of financial barriers to health care has made the lack of a sense of physical safety part of the 'exclusion' experienced by a large part of society. The corollary is the growth of the health care market, which has continued throughout the financial crisis – the pharmaceutical industry has been rated as a 'high-potential foreign direct investment sector' for the coming year.[2] The spirit of optimism that surrounds such well publicised predictions contrasts with the silence that accompanies the experience of absence of care. It is striking to note that, despite the massive insecurity that is being experienced in the face of Poland's health care changes, there has been little discussion or research about what loss of health care safety, in tandem with other social changes, has meant in people's lives.[3] Marketisers cite the growing health care market – the total amount of money spent privately on health care – as reassuring evidence that 'Poles are better off'. A different story is told by national death rates. Mortality among men was 48 percent higher in Poland than in the countries of 'old Europe' in 1990 when communism ended; by 2009 that figure had risen to 58 percent.[4] This increase was largely because health improvements in the intervening period had not been shared equally across the population, but were limited to a relatively narrow affluent social group.[5] Health care changes have been hitting hardest where people need care the most.

This chapter examines the events and processes through which Polish health care changes that centre on privatisation have been pursued over the past two decades – in the face of the profound scepticism, fears and opposition of the public, and despite evidence that casts significant doubt on the extent to which markets have resulted in improved health outcomes, 'efficiency' or access to care. It highlights the complex processes through which marketisers have drawn on long-standing symbolic distinctions between modernity and backwardness both discursively to legitimate the effects of markets, and to promote markets in health care through the creation of a political economy of shame. The chapter identifies key policy decisions through which the gradual but inexorable dismantling of the state-socialist universal system of health care has been occurring and an increasingly privatised system put in its place. It argues that, in order to secure social acquiescence to these strategic changes, reformers have obscured their political implications by deploying disguising discourse when explaining their goals. These discourses overlay globally circulating themes such as 'efficiency' and 'quality', and resonate with the concerns of liberals to achieve a 'modernity' for Poland based on marketisation, which, it is held by unspoken assumption, will ultimately be to the benefit of all. The credibility of this thesis depends on the erasure of the expansion of health care inequalities and the social suffering that the changes have already brought.

Poland's social divisions take centre stage

The generalised optimism of liberal portrayals of social change in Poland was shattered in the wake of the death of the Polish President, when the depth of social divisions was clearly exposed. On April 10, 2010, a Tupolev aircraft carrying ninety-six people, including the President and his wife, crashed into the forest outside the city of Smolensk, killing everyone on board. In addition to the presidential couple, the plane was filled with senior opposition figures and military officials; the death of a national president along with so many of the country's elite in this kind of disaster was a virtually unprecedented event. The aftermath of the accident was critical in its own right. A public outpouring of emotion took place in the immediate wake of the crash. Crowds gathered in the square in front of the Presidential Palace near Warsaw's Old Town, and continued to congregate there for months. While initially the crowds were united in mourning, this unity eventually gave way to repeated incidents of confrontation, which culminated in scenes of anger and near-hysteria centering on the threatened removal from the square of a large crucifix. The episode was swiftly inscribed into the annals of political protest in Poland under a long list of 'struggles for the cross'.[6]

Alongside people who focused on religious symbols and prayer were those who mocked and taunted the religious mourners, and made clear their objection to the increasing presence of holy symbols in public spaces. Adding to the tension were conspiracy theories concerning the cause of the air disaster, which were rife. 'Poles are being cheated, we want the truth' was a common theme. Banners saying '2010: The Perfect Crime' articulated suspicions that the plane had been deliberately brought down. 'Fatherland of mine' the crowd had chanted, 'bathed in blood so many times' (*Ojczyzno ma, tyle razy we krwi skąpana*). Counterposed to this were hostile references to a 'strange tribe', to 'circuses' and 'madmen', and to the antics of '*mohery*' –a disparaging reference to a stereotype of a woman, usually older, religious and prone to wearing a woolly beret.[7] In a context where the mainstream liberal media define Poland's political space in terms of 'victimhood'/backwardness versus 'modernity'/joining a 'post-historical' Europe (Nowak 2011), the mohair beret – imbued with specific age, gender and religious connotations – had acquired the power to signify persons not fully modern or 'European'. The emotions and vociferousness displayed during the clashes were powerful and unexpected enough to prompt extended reflection on the condition of Polish politics, society and state.[8]

The conspiracy theories were widely condemned in the liberal press. For many, the religious mourners were simply beyond the pale; they were 'alien, they are alien, this is not a Poland that I recognise,' said a Warsaw University professor of ethics and liberal feminist.[9]

Yet dismissing conspiracy theories out of hand can mean losing the opportunity for analysis that excessive language of this kind presents, for it may express political fears or social imaginaries that otherwise are unsayable, or that cannot be heard (see Marcus 1999; also Fassin 2008). In this vein, the exchanges that erupted onto the streets of Warsaw can be seen as a political 'coming out'.[10] As a unique political symbol, what the disaster eventually brought to the surface was a mixture of confusion, feelings of powerlessness, threat and anxiety, as well as anger and resentment. Reactions were patterned according to location with respect to social change.

What was fundamentally at issue in the religious manifestations was not religion itself, other commentators suggested, but a mistrust of government and mounting frustration that society itself was being sidelined. Society had come out of the shadows, and the unmediated exchanges that were heard showed to stunned observers that not all was well. According to the sociologist Anna Giza-Poleszczuk, 'most of the "defenders of the cross" are people who feel excluded; on the other side, there are the "happy children of the enlightenment" ... young people from big towns, the kind of people favoured by public opinion pollsters – they always respond "correctly": they are in favour of democracy, freedom, progress, human rights.' But their opposition to the cross was also grounded in emotion, not least in fears of being labelled someone out of the dark ages, in other words – a *ciemnogród*.[11]

An anthropological record of the scenes of mourning over time was provided by the documentary film *Katastrofa*. When asked in an interview what the catastrophe was to which the title referred, the film's director replied that for him, catastrophe signalled the failure of the kind of state whose responsibilities should extend beyond the fetishisation of private property and include taking care of its citizens. By extension of this definition, I propose the term catastrophic citizenship to denote the terms of belonging in this kind of 'failed state', where 'exclusion' can refer not to a minority, but to many, if not most citizens. 'The experience of powerlessness, helplessness, of being orphaned by the state and the elite is the fate of many people,' ... (and) no-one even attempts to talk to them.'[12] Clearly this situation is very far from what was intended when Solidarity first challenged communist rule. Catastrophic citizenship thus also resonates with 'catastrophe' as 'an unexpected ending in a Greek tragedy', which was the original meaning of the term.

While many examples have since been put forward of the way citizens' interests and needs have been neglected, health care arguably is among the most deeply felt of these.[13] As part of a broader context of dependent development in Poland, health care change has led to the loss of health care rights for significant numbers of citizens. By 1989, when communism ended, access to health care – however variable in quality – had become available to everyone virtually free of charge. The policy changes taking place from the early 1990s onwards, coupled with rising pharmaceutical costs, did not fundamentally alter this situation. In 1999, however, a new financing scheme was introduced which effectively resulted in sharply reduced access to medicines and outpatient care. After 1999, a series of unsuccessful attempts were made to privatise hospitals and in 2010, the struggle over hospital privatisation resulted in the enactment of legislation encouraging them to be turned into commercial companies subject to company and commercial law – a turn of events in which the death of the President played an indirect role, as I later show.[14] By 2011, the government was actively pursuing legislation to promote the growth of a private health insurance market. The chapter traces some of these developments, considering how they have affected access to care, how they have been interpreted, concealed and contested, and the implications for understanding citizenship transformation.

A struggle over meaning is pivotal to privatisation – public perceptions have the potential to damage prospects for both profits and electoral success. Convincing public opinion that loss of health care entitlement is right is a challenge, especially where there is mistrust of government, a cultural legacy of scepticism and egalitarianism, and where a large proportion of the population is low-paid. When liberal discourse defines political space in terms of a contrast between backwardness and modernity, this is not so much a way of describing empirical reality but a language for saying what kind of person 'qualifies' in the new Poland, as well as what kind of country the new Poland should be. The question arises as to the purposes served by this pervasive mode of evaluation in the context of health care change. What is the relationship between the ranking of citizens in terms of modernity/backwardness, and loss of access to care? How might this system of representation itself shape access to care? To what extent might such evaluations legitimate a shift from health care as a social right and entitlement, to health care as a liberal – and therefore conditional – right? How does the use of language serve both to differentiate citizenship and mask the unequalising direction of health policy goals? When liberals promote 'modernity', to what extent do they ignore and therefore legitimate their own class interests, and by implication Poland's evolving class system as a whole?[15]

Catastrophic citizenship and dependent development

The development of catastrophic citizenship is closely allied with the way in which Poland has been incorporated into the global political economy since communism came to an end. Rather than engaging in an encounter among equals, Poland was to occupy a subordinate position with respect to a global economy and international power relations effectively dominated by the US. In addition to its prior debt to the IMF and lack of indigenous capital, Poland's subordinate position was also defined symbolically in terms of its difference from a modern West. Since the enlightenment the idea of eastern Europe as backward has held sway. As Larry Wolff has shown, at this time 'the crucial binary opposition between civilization and barbarism assigned Eastern Europe to an ambiguous space, in a condition of backwardness, on a relative scale of development' (Wolff 1994: 127). The Polish sociologist Piotr Sztompka has subscribed to this way of thinking and has articulated a contemporary version of the idea of eastern European backwardness, where the cause is, as he puts it, the 'civilisational incompetence' that is a legacy of communism.

In 1990, the neoliberal direction for change that had been globally formulated for Poland was seized by the country's leaders with both hands. Ironically, Polish politicians were ready to create the markets in health care as part of the early and traumatic shock therapy programme and it was the World Bank which argued instead for sequential reform. Leszek Balcerowicz, the prime local mover in the shock therapy programme, and key decision-maker in the 1999 health financing change, was to write of US health care, that not the market but the state had been to blame for escalating costs (Balcerowicz 1999). 'That's how it is in Poland' a former Minister of Health ruefully remarked. 'Poland is that country, the only one in the world, which loves the Americans always and everywhere, in every situation'.[16]

The persistence of ideas of eastern European inferiority and the way they continue to structure much of public discourse in Europe today has been discussed by Böröcz, who identifies a 'definite geographical pattern to the Europe-wide distribution of moral qualities: goodness is tied to the western (...) parts of the continent' (Böröcz 2006: 129; see also Böröcz 2000). Eastern Europe, some have noted, has been 'semi-orientalised' (Said 1978; see also Syska 2008). The consequences of the symbolic and material asymmetry between the acceding states and the existing EU for structuring the policy-setting process has been described by Jacoby in terms of 'priest and penitent', whereby 'humble CEE countries approached the EU as a sinner approaches a priest, hoping for forgiveness for poor policies and advice on how to come closer to the divine' (quoted in Orenstein 2008: 902). The redemptive pull of 'Westernness' therefore should not be ignored.

All this is not to mention the way the development of eastern European countries as dependent market economies – whereby foreign direct investment (FDI) is attracted by providing a relatively cheap workforce as well as tax breaks for firms (Böröcz and Sarkar 2005; Nölke and Vliegenthart 2009; Bohle and Greskovits 2007) – has itself had significance for health care change. The loss to state finances of potential tax revenue has placed limits on public spending while the lack of ongoing investment in training that is characteristic of FDI lays up future economic problems (Nölke and Vliegenthart 2009; Szelényi and Wilk 2010). Dependent development also introduces social divisions with on the one side, those employed by Western-owned corporations – who enjoy relatively favourable working conditions – and on the other those who are not (Nölke and Vliegenthart 2009).[17] The latter includes people who suffer disproportionately from the restricted social spending that, together with low wages, contributes to the profitability of transnational corporations operating in Poland.

Introducing restrictions to health care access

Major health care change came with a new mechanism of financing laid down in the 1997 Law on Universal Health Insurance, which came into force in January 1999.[18] In place of direct state funding, this introduced a system based on the Bismarckian social insurance model – whereby insurance funds are raised from a compulsory deduction from taxable income. The insurance funds were designed to finance the direct costs of health services to patients through contracts between service providers and purchasers. The latter originally took the form of 16 Regional Sickness Funds (*kasy chorych*), one in each of the new voivodeships, together with one Sickness Fund for uniformed services. The sickness funds were replaced in 2003 by a recentralised National Health Fund (NFZ – *Narodowy Fundusz Zdrowotny*). This performed largely the same functions, and had a branch in each voivodeship. Originally set at 7.5 percent of income and currently standing at 9 percent, the contribution rate was imposed on the intervention of Leszek Balcerowicz, then Minister of Finance. The figure represented a substantial reduction of the level of 10 percent advocated by health care professionals, and the 10–11 percent that had been deemed necessary in earlier bills (Kuszewski and Gericke 2005). Given that the income base from which premiums were deducted was low, with many of those in employment on modest levels of pay and about one-fifth of the working population officially unemployed at the time, the decision resulted in a sharp drop in the public funding available for clinical care (Watson 2006a). The idea was that the gap would be filled by private health care. An opinion poll found that three-quarters of respondents thought that health care provision had been better before the new law (Watson 2006a).

Meanwhile, the establishment of pharmaceutical markets from the early 1990s had significantly increased health care costs. Instead of expanding Polish drug exports as it was said had been intended, the 1994 pharmaceutical industry restructuring programme had led to increased high-cost imports and the domination of the market by transnational pharmaceutical firms. There was ample evidence of shady dealings along the way. For example, the State Monitoring Agency (Najwyższa Izba Kontroli NIK) found that the Polfa Łyszkowice plant, with a nominal value of 4.5 million zloty, had been 'sold' by the local Voivode on behalf of the State Treasury to the German company

Byk Gulden free-of-charge (NIK 2002). This was somewhat short of the 5.5 million price tag mentioned in the press at the time (Rzeczpospolita 1999).

By deploying large promotional budgets, developing strategic interpersonal connections and, increasingly, by using predatory methods involving negative PR, the pharmaceutical companies vigorously pursued sales. Corruption scandals involving public officials and the pharma industry were highlighted in the press. In one case, a Vice Minister of Health was forced to resign when it came to light that the drug Ivabradina had been added to the list of reimbursed medicines shortly after a visit – initially denied – from the producer's medical rep (Jachowicz 2007). In another reported case, the same representative, Robert Pachocki of the firm Servier which also produced the drug Detralex, militated with consecutive Health Ministers to have the generic half-price equivalent Pelethrocin, produced by the drug firm Help, removed from the reimbursement list – at one stage allegedly arriving with a pre-filled in form ready for the health minister to sign along the dotted line (Kosmala 2004). The description offered below of Pachocki, the 'undisputed king of pharmaceutical lobbying' (Jachowicz 2007), indicates the shadowy and influential modus operandi of a successful pharmaceutical sales rep in Poland:

> ... he's good at manipulating people and securing their dependence on him. He might invite someone influential out to lunch. Another time he might ask a well-known professor to provide an evaluation of his drug. He'll willingly fund the lectures of a researcher who is held in high academic regard. But he does it all wearing white gloves. ... He knows all the most important people who can influence the Polish Health system. Everyone knows him too. All the doors to successive Ministers of Health and departmental directors in successive government teams are open to him. He has excellent contacts with members of the parliamentary health commission, and with the journalists that specialise in this field.
>
> (Jachowicz 2007)

By 2008, the proportion of total public spending on health care accounted for by pharmaceuticals had risen to about 15 percent (in the UK the figure is about nine). At the same time, because the levels of drug reimbursement have been lower than in other European countries, the proportion of the costs of pharmaceuticals paid for by people directly is the highest in Europe. Together then, low incomes, increased health care costs and limits to public spending produced large inequalities in access to care (see Table 6.1).

By 2009, according to the results of the Polish Social Diagnosis Survey, just under half of disability pensioner and unwaged households were inhibited from getting the medicine they needed for reasons of cost. Over half had given up the idea of going to the dentist, and about two-thirds of the unwaged were prevented through finances from arranging dentures or from visiting the doctor. Even among those in work, money had prevented 16

Table 6.1 Households not seeking required care for financial reasons 2008–09, by socioeconomic category (percentage)

	Medicines	Dentist	Dentures	Doctor	Tests	Rehab	Hospital
Worker	16	21	26	11	8	17	2
Farmer	22	27	25	16	12	18	2
Self-employed	8	12	24	24	7	13	2
Retired	26	26	29	29	14	24	2
Disability pensioner	44	52	47	47	23	35	3
Unwaged	48	52	65	65	28	39	9

Source: Czapiński and Panek (2009) *Polish Social Diagnosis Survey 2009*, Table 4.7.5, p. 112.

percent from getting the medicine they needed, and had stopped 11 percent from seeing the doctor. Hospitals, in contrast, most of which are unprivatised, remain largely accessible to all.

Health care inequalities and discourses of disguise

One contradiction underlying catastrophic citizenship in Poland is that while theoretically every citizen is still entitled to health care, in practice only some can now obtain it, many having lost access for reasons of finance. How is the contradiction to be squared? This is where the representation of reality in terms of backwardness/modernity comes in. For what it generates is a discourse that disguises the fact that in practice rights have been unequalised. It does this by providing a notional scale against which people can be measured, as a way of determining who is a 'true citizen'.[19] Piotr Sztompka's theory of eastern European 'civilisational incompetence' is an elaborated version of the backwardness/modernity discourse that currently saturates the mainstream liberal media in Poland. According to this theory, civilisational incompetence, which is claimed to be the legacy of real socialism, is the antithesis of the civilisational competence that is the prerequisite for *true modernity* and authentic democracy in post-communist society (original emphasis). Sztompka spells out in detail the criteria which people must meet if they are to develop the mentality that fits them to be 'a full member of a truly modern democracy':

> Four substantive sub-categories of civilisational competence coincide with four main areas of modern, developed society for which they are immediately relevant: *enterprise culture*, indispensable for participation in market economy. Some of its components include: innovative persistence, achievement orientation, individualistic competitiveness, rational calculation, and the like. Second, there is the *civic culture*, indispensable for participation in democratic polity. Some of its components include: political activism, readiness to participate, concern with public issues, rules of law, discipline, respect for opponents, compliance with the majority,

and the like. Third, there is the *discoursive culture* (sic), indispensable for participation in free intellectual flow. Some of its components include: tolerance, open-mindedness, acceptance of diversity and pluralism, scepticism, criticism and the like. And four, there is the *everyday culture*, indispensable for daily existence in advanced, urbanised, technologically saturated and consumer-oriented society. Some of its components include: neatness, cleanliness, orderliness, punctuality, body care, fitness, facility to handle mechanical devices and the like.

(Sztompka 1993: 88–89)[20]

Although the criteria above are defined in terms of mentality, and are meant ideally to apply to post-communist society, they presuppose a level of material and social security more reminiscent of an established Western middle-class. Clearly, they don't draw a line of absolute empirical difference between the qualities of citizens in 'true modernity' and under state socialism. Some of these criteria were met in bold ways before democratisation, political activism and social criticism after all were key to state socialism's demise. Again, many criteria seem detached from the current realities of the lives of people in Poland who are in low paid and insecure jobs, who cannot afford health care, are homeless, unemployed or on a disability pension – and together this encompasses a large part of the population. Affordable health care for many of them is a thing not of the present but of the past. To the extent that the material basis for meeting the criteria for 'true citizenship' is both presupposed and denied in these rules for understanding reality, they operate as a way of translating lack of material resources into a lack of the moral prerequisites for being a 'true citizen' in modern Poland. According to this kind of disguising discourse, people who have lost out in the transition to capitalist democracy, forfeiting access to health care along the way, haven't done so as a result of Poland's position with respect to the international economy, or because of global and government decisions to shrink the workforce and step up income disparities, prioritising private gain over public welfare – but rather because they are intrinsic 'losers' who can't meet the challenges of the new social reality – and who for that reason basically have only themselves to blame.[21]

This normative way of looking at the world asserts a discontinuity between past and present and wipes out much historical and current social context. Specifically, it erases the overriding reality of class creation, since it is based on the presupposition that everyone's experience of transition after communism has been more or less the same. It is part of a memory politics where the past is reduced to a source of individual dysfunction: emancipation from the past being part of what it means to be a 'true citizen'. Furthermore, it does not allow for seeing present experience and memory as inevitably implicated in one another in multiple ways, where neither memory or present experience is prior or able to stand alone (cf. Watson 2006). Not only is experience in the present shaped by memories of the past, as Fassin (2008) among others has noted. But equally, memories of past events are themselves both shaped and reshaped by current interests and experiences – as Edelman (1964, 2001) has also stressed. The multi-valent and variable character of the relationship of memory and present experience, and the strength of alternative moral structures, is illustrated in a 2004 interview with Halina Stolińska, a nurse who had been employed for many years at the health centre at the Nowa Huta steelplant in Kraków.[22] By the time of the interview she had retired, but was working part-time in a clinic in order to supplement her income. She began by describing her time at the steelplant health centre:

> just as I have bad memories of the PRL (Polish People's Republic) period, at the same time – at least in our industrial health group, the Clinic for Occupational Diseases – the care was very good. ... We were together, so to speak. We felt that we were a group that had worked together for a long time, and neither the nurses, nor the doctors, nor the auxiliaries felt that 'oh, that's just an auxiliary, and that's a high-up doctor' ... both the health workers and the patients were happy with (the way things worked). (...) We felt that we were together, not only us health workers, but the health workers and the patients – the ones that were hospitalised here, and the ones that needed our help and came to us. They never left without help. (...)
>
> You know, people are changing now, I don't know where it comes from but they are completely different people, the same people, but completely different. Before there was that unity, that ... solidarity. I'm not just talking about the Solidarity period and the time of martial law, but even earlier, before Solidarity, before 1980 ... Before, they used to talk differently about the patients. (before a patient was) an ill person who has to be helped, you know? ... 'We have to do all we can to help him.' And now – something I never heard before – there are sentences like: 'because patients, they think they're entitled to everything and actually they're not entitled to anything because a hospital, it can only do so much. In a clinic, if a patient doesn't want to queue from five o'clock in the morning to register – well, there are private practices – so what's the problem?' ... The same people ... yet completely different. ... That was a very good period – both for the workers (of the health centre) and for the steelworkers – I'm really ashamed to say it – but there was a time like that in PRL.

Halina Stolińska had been actively opposed to communist rule, putting herself at personal risk in the process, but admitting to good memories of her life in the past gave rise to feelings of shame. She had observed that in such respects doctor–patient relationships were now deteriorating in comparison with what she recalled of her work situation decades before. In her account, doctors had previously felt an imperative to respond to patients' needs by virtue of their humanity, while the empathy and co-operation linking doctors to patients had now grown weak. The attitude of some doctors to medical and financial need was changing to one of indifference. Health care costs for patients who could not afford to pay them, were defined as a 'non-problem'. Her notion of civility was informed by a moral framework that, in contrast to the implications of backwardness/modernity discourse, emphasised equality and solidarity – which she saw as disappearing in the new regime.

The hospitals: secrets, lies and audiotapes

How then has disguising discourse been used to shape acquiescence to health policy change? In this section, I consider this question in relation to hospital privatisation. With the 1999 health reform legislation it became technically possible for hospitals to privatise. Nevertheless, they remain largely public and accessible, accounting for close to one half of public spending on health care.[23] As such, they are a prime target for the expansion of markets in health care (Goc and Gerczyk 2011). In 2000, the World Bank had commissioned a report from Gorden Greenshields, staunch advocate of the discredited Private Financing Initiative (PFI) in the British NHS.[24] The task was to define 'the goals and strategies for appropriate privatization in in-patient hospital care in Poland' (Greenshields 2000). The report pointed to what it saw as the wrong thinking that the idea of privatisation provoked: 'Some read into the word a plot to create/restore a completely free market, with overtones of "dog eat dog", "exploitation of the weakest" and "survival of the fittest" … Still others are provoked by the term because they see it as an attack on the ideals they cherish. "Public" to them denotes brotherhood, sharing, and community, and they mistakenly interpret "private" to mean the negation of these important values' (p. 20). One of the conclusions was that integral to any strategy for hospital privatisation was a battle for hearts and minds.

Given the strength of antipathy to privatisation, the need to win elections and to accommodate the pressures exerted by corporations, the government feinted non-privatisation. What was said to be planned was the 'commercialisation' of hospitals instead. Through commercialisation, efficiency would be increased. Debt played a key role in this case of 'policy in search of a rationale' (Pollock et al. 2002), since it was presented as incontrovertible evidence of inefficiency, proof that public hospitals could not manage their funds. Emphasis on the debt-inefficiency nexus masked the fact that hospitals were systematically underfinanced. For figures clearly showed that the limits to funding introduced in 1999 had resulted in contractual rates of payment to hospitals that were significantly less than the cost of services in practice.[25] Hospitals had frequently borrowed to make good those funding shortfalls. Interest rates on earlier debts, court costs and losses to debt collectors – who were entitled to remove life-saving hospital equipment and to access hospital bank accounts – aggravated the situation. Debt collecting firms and debt purchasing firms, on the other hand, experienced a boom.[26] Yet at the same time government did nothing following official notification of pharmaceutical companies' widespread practice of privatising hospital and NFZ resources, that is to say, drawing on them without compensation, in order to run clinical trials in hospitals as a way of upping sales (cf. NIK 2010).[27]

Events during the 2007 election campaign appeared to confirm people's worst fears. During the campaign, health care issues played a prominent role. The Anti-Corruption Bureau (*Centralne Biuro Anti-Korupcyjne* – CBA), the creation of the Law and Justice (PiS) Party then in power, had released secretly recorded tapes of a conversation between a Civic Platform Party parliamentarian, Beata Sawicka, and a CBA official posing as a businessman. The tapes caused a furore:

> 'I have a group of people,' Sawicka was caught on tape as saying, 'it's not a large group of people, because there's three of us ... who have, make, you know, the law and so on ... but most of all who have enormous knowledge about what's going to happen in the future, that's to say the privatisation of parts of the health service ... There's going to be a rationalisation of the hospital network, the local authorities are going to get rid of the assets, that's to say they're going to sell them and turn hospitals into commercial companies ... Well as everyone knows – medicine's going to be private, hospitals are going to be private ... What's it going to start from? From having to submit a tender for a hospital and then having to buy it ... But if ... let's say, you turn a hospital or a clinic into a commercial company, then you simply take over the building, and the structure, and the people. The people with a head start will be the ones in the know (quoted in Misiak 2008).
>
> Just wait until we've won the elections, that's when we'll really start doing the business (*to do piero będziemy kręcić lody*) (quoted in Kowalski 2007).

Sawicka was expelled from the Civic Platform and her Party promised not to privatise hospitals, but an investigation into the affair was never carried out. Instead, the Party and the mainstream press 'shrieked out' modernity versus anachronism as the electoral alternatives, and the Civic Platform won (Nowak 2011: 2). Shortly after the election, the government instituted high profile social consultations on health care change, producing an agreement symbolising that dialogue had taken place, but which bore absolutely no relation to the legislation subsequently proposed. This raised questions as to what had occurred behind the scenes to radically transform policy direction in the meantime. According to the new proposals, the law was to make it compulsory for all hospitals – most of which were still independently functioning units under local authority management – to become businesses, thus opening the way for their sale. The new proposals were put to Parliament in the form of a members', not a government, bill – thus obviating the statutory requirement for social consultation. Most of the organisations who were not consulted were against the compulsory commercialisation of hospitals, and had indicated this at a meeting with the President (Cichocka 2008).[28]

The Prime Minister insisted that turning hospitals into businesses owned by local authorities was in fact communalisation, not privatisation at all (Gazeta Prawna 2008). The healthworkers' unions argued that commercialisation meant an open door to privatisation, saying that it would bring a worsening of living conditions for both workers and patients, and would bring further social divisions and worse access to health care for the poor. Approximately one month later, the President used his powers to veto the bill.

The death of the President in the Smolensk air crash was followed by early elections. Health care reform was the unspoken campaign issue, not least because during the election the word 'privatisation' was judicially banned. The Civic Platform party obtained a court ruling to the effect that hospital privatisation could not be legally imputed to them as a goal. The opposing Law and Justice Party successfully appealed, whereupon the Civic Platform returned to court to have the original ruling upheld. The subsequent election of a new President from the same Party as the one in government marked a turning point in the prospects for privatisation. It meant that the government was free to move forward untrammelled by countervailing Presidential powers; a law encouraging hospital commercialisation was passed soon afterwards. Barely a year had elapsed when a telegram released by Wikileaks was made public. It gave an account of a meeting between Lee Feinstein, then the US Ambassador, and Jan Bielecki, chief of the Prime Minister's Economic Office and former premier. The meeting had taken place in January 2010, three months before Smolensk. 'Poles, according to Bielecki, are skeptical of a pure, European-style public sector' read the Ambassador's telegram. 'He anticipates privatization of some healthcare assets. Bielecki thinks that there are promising opportunities for U.S. investors with healthcare experience and that U.S. leadership could help along the partial privatization process already in progress.'[29] 'This telegram proves that the government has been thinking of privatisation all along. The Civic Platform officially denies it,' said Marek Balicki, a former Health Minister, 'but is doing something completely different behind the scenes. Worse, it's already happening. It's happened in Kostrzyn on Oder, and now it's happening in Kielce. The privatisation of other places is probably only a matter of time.'[30]

Private health insurance and the political economy of shame

At the twentieth jubilee of the Economic Forum held in Krynica in October 2010, health ministers put forward plans to open the way for competition among payers in the health care system. In this, they drew heavily on backwardness/modernity discourse. The Minister of Health emphasised repeatedly that the bill which had been prepared was motivated by a desire to 'civilise' private expenditure on health care: 'we must propose something that will take up the 20–30 milliard zloty we currently spend on health care outside of the NFZ,' she stressed (Kuropaś 2010). The Vice-Minister of Health described as 'barbaric' out-of pocket payments where actual money changed hands: 'The form of payment where I come and pay for a procedure, is in my opinion a very barbaric form of financing health care, completely out of keeping with the fact that we are now in the 21st century.'[31] Another speaker, Łukasz Zalicki from Ernst & Young, said that an effective health system should be as competitive as possible. 'What it's all about is transforming the current very primitive method of purchasing medical services into more civilised instruments, that is, insurance policies ... (which) are simply a more modern way of our spending the same money (as direct private payments now),' he explained in a subsequent interview (Puls Medyczny 2010).

This example serves as an illustration of the way health care transformation in Poland involves the attempt to mobilise backwardness/modernity discourse in order to create a political economy of shame.[32] It is a political economy of shame because efforts are made to graft feelings of shame and the fear of being shamed as a result of being labelled backward, onto the pushing of markets in health care. The implicit threat is that people who fail to purchase health insurance will be deemed inferior, not as a result of their limited finances, but because they don't meet the required standards of 'true' citizenship. Framing the intentions of the bill in cultural rather than financial terms masked the fact that the central purpose of the proposed law was to serve the material interests of health insurance firms. The bill had been drawn up with the help of the health insurance industry, to the exclusion of input from social organisations (Zdrowie Publiczne 2011).[33] Its purpose was not to make private health insurance legal, which it already was, but to make it more popular – and therefore profitable – by making state budget resources available to promote the industry – primarily through the introduction of tax relief. Thus, according to one health insurance website: 'every paragraph of the Bill serves the development of private health insurance, from the definitions, classifications and regulations concerning the interface of public and private money, to the clear inclusion of occupational health under the heading of insurance, to possible tax exemptions.'[34] Although the bill was widely criticised and eventually stalled because the Ministry of Finance could not permit it given current levels of budget deficit, the PR campaigns that were waged remain part of a longer-term effort to change public perceptions so that private health insurance can eventually be introduced as part of a new health care system.

In addition to framing the introduction of private health insurance in terms of a civilising mission, the argument also included misleading interpretations both of public data and privately commissioned research. Equating 'all private health care payments' with 'fees for medical service', whereby transformation into health insurance payments was all that was required, also helped construct the aim of the Bill in terms of cultural conversion, veiling the possibility that private interests might be at stake. It helped create the 'cultural issue' said to be involved. For example, the reality is that over half of the private spending which the Vice-Minister of Health had termed 'barbaric', over 16 milliard zloty, was accounted for by people's direct expenditure on pharmaceuticals; that is to say, the result of high costs, low levels of drug reimbursement, the vigorous pursuit of increased sales by pharmaceutical firms, not to mention pro-industry pressures exerted by the European Union (2009 figures, see Goc and Gerczyk 2011: 7).[35]

Also excluded from the PR discussions were the findings of research commissioned not long before by Ernst & Young. The study had been designed to show whether the introduction of competition among third-party-payers in Polish health care would increase the efficiency of the system, and had found no evidence that it would.[36] A methodology had been devised to compare 29 countries and found that some single-payer system countries are more efficient than some countries with a multi-payer system. Correlations were between input and outcome on the one hand using investment indicators – such as percentage of GDP, number of hospital beds, personnel, and outcome indicators such as disability-free life expectancy, infant mortality rates, and the Eurohealth consumer index. The research showed that 'there are countries that have a single payer that are more efficient than some countries where there is competition – Poland came out quite well.'[37]

Ernst & Young rejected the report because they were 'frightened that it could be interpreted that if the study showed that competition doesn't improve, that monopoly is better. … .You could see that whether there is a single payer or multiple payers doesn't make much difference … It could have been used for completely the wrong reason, so to speak … It was not the right time to present something like that.' Ernst & Young therefore redefined the terms of reference of the research. 'So we changed it … the question was changed to: what conditions have to be met if competition is to have the desired effects?' The report was published in September 2010 (Więckowska 2010). It advocated a gradually increasing role for private health insurers: 'Bringing in a (private health insurance) system straight away, Poles would feel cheated again – Just as they didn't understand the pension system, and they still don't, there's still not that much dissatisfaction with it because the first payments in the new (pension) system are only just coming through now.'[38] Given the history behind the report, the press release which Ernst & Young issued to accompany its publication was worthy of note. 'The National Health Fund must have competition,' ran the headline as if the original study had never been carried out. 'Competition between payers' it continued, 'is a necessary condition for improving the efficiency of the Polish health care system.'[39]

Concluding remarks

The conspiracy theories and the opposing anti-church sentiments that were expressed in the vociferous aftermath of the death of the president have put into question dominant liberal discourses of political transformation in Poland, whereby, theoretically, marketising changes benefit all. Increased social inequalities have been an integral feature of the formation of dependent capitalism in Poland, where global market agendas have been ascendant. The process of policy-making has undergone privatisation and informalisation, and health care is no exception to this (Wedel 2010). The physical and psychic vulnerabilities to which the health care changes have given rise, coupled with the suspicion – fuelled by periodic leaks – that damaging deals are being done behind closed doors, have contributed to the underlying sense of paranoia and threat. For far from addressing social need, the orientation of successive governments has been towards securing social acquiescence for marketising policies which will further deepen inequalities. An indispensable part of this exercise have been discourses of disguise.

Establishing backwardness/modernity as the key terms in which the space of transformation in Poland is to be defined, plays a central role in disguising discourse. It provides a potent language in terms of which citizens can be differentiated from each other and defined as inherently unequal, thereby diverting perception away from the unequalising goals of political change. It allows lack of health care to be read as a sign of inherent inferiority – of personal failure rather than a symptom of 'catastrophic citizenship' and a 'failed state'. As a way of locating blame for lack of health care with those who experience disadvantage, backwardness/modernity discourse therefore serves to mask the power relations through which that health care disadvantage has been produced.

The political spin surrounding the promotion of private health insurance illustrates how backwardness/modernity discourse has been used as a form of implicit intimidation in the pursuit of policies that urgently serve particular interests and that by the same token – and as is also clear from the US – will put new health care inequalities in place. Since the language of backwardness versus modernity justifies wealth-poverty differences, it helps keep them in place. As a form of intimidation, it contributes to 'a structural censorship (...) that condemns the occupants of dominated positions either to silence or shocking outspokenness' (Bourdieu 1991: 138). It defines who counts as a citizen in Poland, and who can be ridiculed or ignored. As an instance of 'symbolic violence', the violence embodied in concepts, language and symbolic systems designed to obscure unspoken conditions of rule (Bourdieu and Passeron 1977), this form of language is a significant part of the process of class-creation that has been taking place in Poland, amongst others, through health care change.

Notes

1 This chapter draws on research funded by the British Academy. Thanks to Michele Rivkin-Fish for helpful comments.
2 Pawełkowska, A. (2011) 'Poland the 6th most attractive investment destination in the world'. http://washington.trade.gov.pl/en/aktualnosci/article/a,18970.html
3 An exception is the work of Hanna Palska (2002). See also Watson (2006a, 2006b).
4 World Health Organization, 'Health For All' Database.
5 *Polish Demographic Yearbook* data.

6 In the words of one commentator: 'Tylko pod krzyżem, tylko pod tym znakiem, Polska jest Polską, a Polak Polakiem ... Who doesn't know that famous couplet, which in simple and clear words describes the ageless phenomenon of attachment to the traditions of Polish culture founded on Christianity. That is why among other things, the partitioning forces, the Germans and the Soviets during World War II, and after the war, the communists, all fought the cross. Today it's the "camp of progress and democracy" that is fighting the cross' (Jackowski 2011).

7 The liberal press, notably *Gazeta Wyborcza*, which has the largest circulation of any daily newspaper in Poland, has played a significant role in circulating some of the disparaging attitudes heard in the crowd.

8 'Before the catastrophe, one [might] have been forgiven for thinking that the sense of stabilisation, the relatively mild experience of financial crisis, and general satisfaction with the effects of entry to the European Union would lessen social conflicts and sharp political divisions. But after 10 April, and especially after the Presidential elections and the "struggle for the cross", different interpretations have started to appear which emphasise the depth of the divisions.' Aleksander Smolar, Introduction to the discussion held at the Stefan Batory Foundation in Warsaw on April 7, 2011: *Polska po katastrofie. Państwo-społeczeństwo-polityka*, www.batory.org.pl/debaty/2011 0407.htm

9 Professor Magdalena Środa during the panel discussion: *Nieudane Państwo? Co Katastrofa Smoleńska Mówi o Polskiej Wspólnocie*. www.artmuseum.pl/wideo.php? l=0&id=katastrofa

10 This was a phrase used by Artur Żmijewski, director of the film *Katastrofa*.

11 Anna Giza-Poleszczuk in Sommer (2010).

12 *Ibid.*

13 Giza-Poleszczuk gives as examples government rules that require small business owners to pay VAT up front before invoices are settled, and official attitudes to the rural population who are left to their own devices, until they 'just die out' (Sommer 2010).

14 That is, those hospitals owned by local authorities. The law doesn't apply to teaching hospitals.

15 Elena Gapova has critiqued the role of Belorus liberals in these terms when they promote 'democracy' (Gapova 2004).

16 Interview carried out on April 23, 2009.

17 The employment conditions offered by transnational firms often include the provision of prepaid medical packages.

18 This law was subjected to legal challenge, scrapped as unconstitutional and updated in 2003.

19 The intended parallel here is with debates over the way New World Indians should be treated in the evolving colonial system. Stuart Hall (1995) describes how the notion of 'true men' was evoked in order to define which natives could not be enslaved – thereby justifying the enslavement of the rest.

20 The Hungarian sociologist Zsusza Ferge has called Sztompka's theory 'malevolent' (Ferge 2008).

21 A recent article by an academic at the Warsaw School of Economics, a number of whose academics have close links with Ernst & Young, recently quoted Sztompka's paper at length in order to draw a connection between Poland's failure to make more economic progress and the country's supposed cultural deficiencies (Murdoch 2009).

22 Interview carried out on January 24, 2004. Halina Stolińska is a pseudonym.

23 By 2007 there were 170 private hospitals representing approximately 23 percent of non-psychiatric hospitals in Poland, accounting for fewer than 6 percent of hospital beds (Polish Ministry of Health Statistical Yearbook data). Similarly, shortfalls in health care provision did not lead to a surge in private health insurance. By 2010, Poland's private health insurance market was worth only about 160 million zloty, with fewer than 50,000 people in possession of an individual health insurance policy (PIU 2011: 11).

24 The high cost of PFI was originally signalled by Allyson Pollock and colleagues (see, for example, Pollock et al. 2002).
25 For example, a 2008 survey of psychiatric in-patient care found that contracts with the NFZ in general covered between 60 and 80 percent of costs. In 2006–07, the daily rate paid by the NFZ per person and per day in a psychiatric ward stood at 78 and 84 zloty, respectively, while in the Lubiąż hospital, for example, the average cost per person and per day was 125.11 and 145.5 zloty, respectively. This resulted in losses to the hospital of 1.55 million zloty in 2005, 2.41 million zloty in 2006, and 973,700 zloty in the first half of 2007 (Najwyższa Izba Kontroli 2008: 36).
26 Gabriel Pietrasik, then Chair of the National Debt Collectors' Council, pointed out that in the talks leading up to the decision of the Constitutional Tribunal on January 9, 2007, Council suggestions that equipment vital to saving patient life should be excluded from what was collected were explicitly rejected by the Tribunal (Stankiewicz 2007).
27 Pharmaceutical companies have been active in recruiting medical experts to run trials as a way of boosting sales: 'Those trials mean a pile of money, a million, two. The doctor in charge gets a huge payment. … The problem is that if you look more closely the drug may have been tested before – not once, but 800 times … The drug gets tested, the specialists earn legally, let's say 50,000 a month. Everyone's happy … The drug reaches the consciousness of patients and suddenly it's pre-scribed more frequently than it was. That's the way it seems to go' (Interview with Andrzej Sośnierz, former NFZ chief; Majewski and Reszka 2011).
28 'Union leaders appeal to the president to veto health laws', November 24, 2008. www.polskieradio.pl/iar/wiadomosci/artykul76723.html
29 'Former PM Bielecki on U.S.–Poland Economic', created 2010-01-21 11:20; released 2011-08–30, 01:44. http://wikileaks.org/cable/2010/01/10WARSAW48.html
30 *Ibid.*
31 www.orange.pl/kid,4000000150,id,4000277478,title,MZ-dodatkowe-ubezpieczenia-i-konkurencja-dla-NFZ,article.html
32 This is a kind of negative counterpart to the 'political economy of hope', which Rose (2006) has described as being a characteristic of biological citizenship in advanced Western societies.
33 'I like Kopacz (then the Health Minister)' said one informant linked with the health insurance industry. 'She goes to the industry and says: "I have a proposal for legislation – tell me what you don't like about it".'
34 *Czy Ustawa o Dodatkowych Ubezpieczeniach Zdrowotnych Jest Potrzebna?*, www.med icapolska.pl/ubezpieczenie-zdrowotne/czy-ustawa-o-dodatkowych-ubezpieczeniach-zdrowotnych-jest-potrzebna
35 Taking account also of the fact that dental care and prepaid health care packages represent a further 5 million zloty of private expenditure, the amount spent on direct payment of fees for medical service becomes smaller still.
36 This account is closely based on an insider interview dated November 11, 2010.
37 *Ibid.*
38 *Ibid.*
39 See, for example, www.bankier.pl/wiadomosc/Ernst-Young-NFZ-musi-miec-kon-kurencje-2210103.html

References

Balcerowicz, L. (1999) Składka na Zdrowie, in *Państwo w Przebudowie*, Kraków: Znak.
Bohle, D. and Greskovits, B. (2007) 'Neoliberalism, embedded neoliberalism and neocorporatism: towards transnational capitalism in Central-Eastern Europe', *West European Politics*, 30(3): 443–66.

Bourdieu, P. (1991) *Language and Symbolic Power*, Cambridge, MA: Harvard University Press.

Bourdieu, P. and Passeron, J.-C. (1977[1990]) *Reproduction in Education, Society and Culture*, trans. L. Wacquant, London: Sage.

Böröcz, J. (2000) 'The fox and the raven: the European Union and Hungary renegotiate the margins of "Europe"', *Comparative Studies in Society and History*, 42(4): 847–75.

——(2006) 'Goodness is elsewhere: the rule of European difference', *Comparative Studies in Society and History*, 48(1): 110–37.

Böröcz, J. and Sarkar, M. (2005) 'What is Europe?', *International Sociology*, 20(2): 153–73.

Cichocka, E. (2008) 'Bez Referendum w Sprawie Prywatyzacji Szpitali', *Gazeta Wyborcza*, October 29.

Czapiński, J. and Panek, T. (eds) (2009) *Polish Social Diagnosis Survey 2009*, Warszawa: Rada Minitoringu Społecznego.

Edelman, M. (1964[1985]) *The Symbolic Uses of Politics*, Urbana, IL: University of Illinois Press.

——(2001) *The Politics of Misinformation*, Cambridge: Cambridge University Press.

Fassin, D. (2008) 'The embodied past. From paranoid style to politics of memory in South Africa', *Social Anthropology*, 16(3): 312–28.

Ferge, Zs. (2008) 'Is there a specific East–Central European welfare culture?' in W. Van Oorschot, M. Opielka and B. Pfau-Effinger (eds) *Culture and Welfare State: Values and Social Policy in Comparative Perspective*, London: Edward Elgar.

Gapova, E. (2004) 'The nation in between; or, why intellectuals do things with words', in Forrester, S., Zaborowska, M.J. and Gapova, E. (eds) *Communist Cultures Through an East–West Gaze*, Bloomington, IN: Indiana University Press.

Gazeta Prawna (2008) 'Tusk: Nie Prywatyzacja, a Komunalizacja Szpitali', *Gazeta Prawna*, May 9. http://praca.gazetaprawna.pl/artykuly/17010,tusk_nie_prywatyzacja_a_komunalizacja_szpitali.html

Goc, S. and Gerczyk, I. (2011) *Jak Zagospodarować Rynek Ubezpieczeń w Polsce?* Warsawa: Deloitte Polska.

Greenshields, G. (2000) *Task 5: Define the Goals and Strategies of Appropriate Privatization of In-Patient Hospital Care in Poland*, Warrington, UK: Bywater Consulting.

Hall, S. (1995) 'The West and the rest: discourse and power', in S. Hall, D. Held, D. Hubert and K. Thompson (eds), *Modernity: An Introduction to Modern Societies*, Cambridge: Polity Press.

Jackowski, J.C. (2011) '6 Sekund, Ktore Wstrząsnęły Polakami', *Nasz Dziennik*, 83, 9–10 April. www.naszdziennik.pl/index.php?dat=20110409&typ=re&id=re36.txt

Jachowicz, J. (2007) 'Robert Pachocki – Szara Eminencja Rynku Leków', *Dziennik.pl*, November 23. http://wiadomosci.dziennik.pl/polityka/artykuly/158453,robert-pachocki-szara-eminencja-rynku-lekow.html

Kosmala, I. (2004) 'Prochy Marne', *NIE*, 39: 9. www.nie.com.pl/art4261.htm

Kowalski, A. (2007) 'Posłanka PO: W politykę sie nie mieszajcie, tylko kasę dajcie. Kręcenie lodów na prywatyzacji szpitali', *Nasz Dziennik*, 243, October 17. www.naszdziennik.pl/index.php?typ=po&dat=20071017&id=po81.txt

Kuropaś, D. (2010) 'Dodatkowe Ubezpieczenia Zdrowotne: Ten Projekt Jest Wyzwaniem Politycznym', *Rynek Zdrowia*, October 21. www.rynekzdrowia.pl/Ubezpieczenia-zdrowotne/Dodatkowe-ubezpieczenia-zdrowotne-ten-projekt-jest-wyzwaniem-polityczn ym,102919,4.html

Kuszewski, K. and Gericke, C. (2005) *Poland, Health Systems in Transition*, 7: 5, Copenhagen: WHOEuro.

Majewski, M. and Reszka, P. (2011) 'Lekarz to Zawód, a Zawód to Pieniądze', *Rzeczpospolita*, May 21–22, P2–P3.

Marcus, G.E. (1999) 'Introduction: the paranoid style now', in G. Marcus (ed.) *Paranoia Within Reason. A Casebook on Conspiracy as Explanation*, Chicago, IL: Chicago University Press.

Misiak, L. (2008) 'Grupa Rozgrywająca Szpitale', *Gazeta Polska*. http://wiadomosci.onet.pl/1463341,2677,1,1,grupa_rozgrywajaca_szpitale,kioskart.html

Murdoch, A. (2009) 'How much culture is there in corruption? Some thoughts on transformation-cum-collective culture shock in post-communist Poland', *Journal of Intercultural Management*, 1(1): 42–63.

NIK (2002) *Informacja o Wynikach Kontroli Prywatyzacji Branży Farmaceutycznej*, Warszawa: Najwyższa Izba Kontroli.

——(2008) *Informacja o Wynikach Kontroli Funkcjonowania Opieki Psychiatrycznej, Ze Szczególnym Uwzględnieniem Opieki Stacjonarnej*, Wrocław: Najwyższa Izba Kontroli, Delegatura We Wrocławiu.

——(2010) *Informacja o Wynikach Kontroli Realizacji Zakupów Sprzętu Medycznego i Leków przez Szpitale Kliniczne oraz Finansowania przez Dostawców Różnych Sfer Działalności tych Szpitali, w tym Dotyczących Badań Klinicznych*, Katowice: Najwyższa Izba Kontroli, Delegatura w Katowicach.

Nowak, A. (2011) 'From memory clashes to a general battle: the battle for Smoleńsk/Katyń', *East European Memory Studies*, 6: 1–4.

Nölke, A. and Vliegenthart, A. (2009) 'Enlarging the varieties of capitalism: the emergence of dependent market economies in East Central Europe', *World Politics*, 61(4): 670–702.

Orenstein, M. A. (2008) 'Out-liberalizing the EU: pension privatization in Central and Eastern Europe', *Journal of European Public Policy*, 15(6): 899–917.

Palska, M. (2002) *Bieda i Dostatek: O Nowych Stylach Życia w Polsce Końca Lat Dziewięcdziesiątych*. Warsaw: IFiS PAN.

PIU (2011) *Rola Prywatnych Ubezpieczeń w Systemie Ochrony Zdrowia. Jak Wpływają na Dostęp do Świadczeń, Innowacji i Leków – Kluczowe Tezy i Rekomendacje*, Warszawa: PIU.

Pollock, A.M., Shaoul, J. and Vickers, N. (2002) 'Private finance and "value for money" in NHS hospitals: a policy in search of a rationale?' *BMJ*, 324: 1205, doi: 10.1136/bmj.324.7347.1205.

Rose, N. (2006) 'Biological citizenship', in *The Politics of Life Itself: Biomedicine, Power, and Subjectivity in the Twenty-First Century*, Princeton, NJ: Princeton University Press.

Rzeczpospolita (1999) 'Niemcy Kupili Udziały w Polfie Łyszkowice', *Rzeczpospolita*, February 11. http://archiwum.rp.pl/artykul/213696_Niemcy_kupili_udziały_w_Polfie_Lyszkowice.html

Said, E. (1978) *Orientalism*, Harmondsworth: Penguin.

Sommer, M. (2010) 'Fajni ludzie pod krzyżem,' *Rzeczpospolita*, August 16. www.rp.pl/artykul/523149.html

Stankiewicz, M. (2007) 'Trybunał Strzela Szpitalom w Piętę', *Gazeta Lekarska*, 2. www.gazetalekarska.pl/res/img/img/nil/gazeta/n200702.pdf

Syska, A. (2008) 'Eastern Europe in the making of US identity', PhD thesis, St Louis University, Missouri, USA.

Sztompka, P. (1993) 'Civilizational incompetence: the trap of post-communist societies', *Zeitschrift für Soziologie*, 22(2): 85–95.

Puls Medyczny (2010) 'To Pacjent Powinien Wybierać', *Puls Medycyny*, 16. www.pulsmedycyny.com.pl/index/archiwum/13698,pacjent,powinien,wybiera%C4%87.html

Szelényi, I. and Wilk, K. (2010) 'From socialist workfare to capitalist welfare state', in *The Oxford Handbook of Comparative Institutional Analysis*, Oxford: Oxford University Press.

Watson, P. (2006a) 'Unequalizing citizenship: the politics of Poland's health care change', *Sociology*, 40(6): 1079–1096.

——(2006b) 'Stress and social change in Poland', *Health and Place*, 12: 372–82.

Wedel, J. (2010) *Shadow Elite: How the World's New Power Brokers Undermine Democracy, Government and the Free Market*, New York: Basic Books.

Więckowska, B. (2010) *Konkurencja Między Płatnikami w Bazowym Systemie Zabezpieczenia Zdrowotnego*, Warszawa: Ernst & Young.

Wolff, L. (1994) *Inventing Eastern Europe. The Map of Civilisation on the Mind of the Enlightenment*, Stanford, CA: Stanford University Press.

Zdrowie Publiczne (2011) 'Ostry Sprzeciw Partnerów Społecznych Przeciw Ustawie o Dodatkowym Ubezpieczeniu Zdrowotnym', *Zdrowie Publiczne*, June 10. www.zdro wie-publiczne.com.pl/wiadomosc_ostry-sprzeciw-partnerow-spolecznych-przeciw-ustawie-o-dodatkowym-ubezpieczeniu-zdrowotnym-325.html

7 The making of health care policy in contemporary Hungary[1]

Terry Cox and Sandor Gallai

Introduction

This chapter reviews the main measures introduced by successive governments since 1990 to bring about a transformation of the health care system in post-communist Hungary. It lays special emphasis on changes to the financing of health care; the issue of citizen and interest group participation; and the ownership of hospitals. A recurrent theme in the making of health policy has been its highly contested nature and the perceived ineffectiveness of several of the measures that have been introduced. The paper explores this problem through an analysis of key characteristics of the Hungarian polity as it has emerged since 1990, and the relations between policy actors in the making of health policy in Hungary. Drawing on documentary and interview-based research with a wide range of different state and social actors, including government ministers, civil servants, political parties, consultants and representatives of doctors and other health care workers, the chapter examines debates and competition between them in their attempts to influence policy-making.

Twenty-two years after the regime change in Hungary, the situation of the health sector is rather ambiguous. On one hand, a series of institutional reforms has resulted in major changes: health care has been opened up to the market, to the influence of globalisation on its economy, and to private ownership. The roles of purchasing, service provision and financing have been separated; regulatory, monitoring and supervisory bodies are in place; a new system of financing has been established; patients' rights have been enacted; consultative bodies have been set up; and representation of professional and patient organisations has been institutionalised. On the other hand, the management of the health sector and the operation of health institutions are subject to widespread criticism from health professionals and the public alike. Discontent has focused in particular on poor levels of public health; a limited emphasis on health promotion and the prevention of illness; extensive hospitalisation and growing waiting lists; corruption; and the apparent failure of successive post-communist governments to resolve the key issues of finance and ownership. In certain areas, such as gynaecology, dentistry and kidney dialysis centres, private service providers play an outstanding role, while private owners and operators either have remained insignificant or have failed entirely in the running of hospitals. What is more, recent decisions suggest that the ownership of a wide range of health institutions will be transferred from the municipal governments to the central government and its county representatives.

The interconnected issues of finance and privatisation have been particularly intractable. For most of the period since the regime change, the provision of health care has been in deficit, and attempts to reduce the deficit have entailed severe cuts in expenditure that have been extremely unpopular. Between 1990 and 2002, the central budget had to pay HUF 30–80 billion annually to cover the deficit of the Health Insurance Fund (HIF), and after 2002 the deficit increased considerably to a figure in excess of HUF 300 billion. Only in 2006–07 did government policies succeed in removing the deficit so that the balance of the Fund turned into a slight surplus for the first time. This effective deficit reduction was achieved through bureaucratic control mechanisms and the weakening of incumbent interests in the sector. How-ever, the reform package also involved severe cuts in health expenditures.[2] The Hungarian electorate tends to have strong feelings on health issues and is generally opposed to cuts in public health expenditure. This has posed a serious dilemma for successive governments. While higher revenues could have reduced the size of the cuts, the already high levels of taxation did not make a significant increase of health contributions possible politically. Thus governments generally have avoided painful interventions unless budgetary constraints left no room for escape.

In this context, privatisation of health services has been seen by government at national and local levels as an important part of a solution to the problem of financing the system and, in theory, it could have provided the best pos-sibilities specifically for generating revenues. Successive governments have made attempts to privatise hospitals and other health care institutions, but in the fierce bipartisan context of a strongly polarised party system until the 2010 elections, this has not been feasible politically. While private actors are already present in the health sector, under the prevailing financial regulations neither contracting out further services nor privatising entire health institutions has been regarded as an attractive option.

In 2010, the Hungarian Civic Union (Fidesz) won a major electoral victory and obtained a qualified two-thirds majority in parliament. As a result, the current government enjoys nearly unlimited legal freedom in the formulation of health policy. However, the fierce public opposition to privatisation and co-payment during the previous government's term has made it politically difficult for Fidesz to incorporate such ideas into its policy mix. In fact, the new government intends to tackle the country's financial difficulties partly by reinforcing the role of the state in delivering public services. Thus the first drafts of a new bill on local government advocate that responsibility for secondary and tertiary care and the ownership of the respective institutions should belong to the state.

In this chapter, we seek to understand the political background that explains the dilemmas and contradictions involved in the making of health policy in contemporary Hungary. In the first section, we briefly describe the legacy of the communist-period health care system. We then examine in turn the key features of the reformed post-communist political system and the institutional framework in health care, before examining the story of privatisation reform in the area of health policy. The final section discusses some of the key reasons for the failure of successive governments to develop a clear regulatory framework for the role of private ownership in the provision of health care, and attempts to explain the most recent shift towards an unusually extensive role for the government.

The legacy of the previous system

The communist regime in Hungary, as elsewhere, was characterised by centralised, concentrated power and extensive state intervention. In the health sector, the state was not simply the owner of health institutions and facilities, but also the manager, provider and financer of their services (Gaál 2004: 6). The Constitution of 1949 declared health to be one of the fundamental rights of citizens, and the state was put in charge of providing health services that were in principle accessible to all citizens and free at the point of use. In practice, however, the quality of services available to citizens depended on many factors, including special facilities for elite members, informal connections, 'under-the-table' payments and gratuities, which all distorted the principle of equality. The legal environment did not recognise the concept of patients' rights, and it also failed to address ethical issues.[3]

Then, in the 1980s, there were a number of important changes in the health sector that were in line with the general developments of the country associated with the market reforms of the New Economic Mechanism. In Hungary, uniquely in the region, the beginnings of the introduction of a market mechanism and the legalisation of private ownership and entrepreneurship were introduced by the communist state and thus preceded the political transformation of 1989–90 (Gallai 2009: 186–7). Specifically in relation to health care, the communist political leadership permitted part-time private practices for specialists such as dentists, dermatologists, urologists and gynaecologists. With the new forms of service provision, a dual structure emerged where public services continued to dominate the sector, but private services were also beginning to expand. Policy management in the health sector was still based on central rule, and professional interest groups were tightly controlled. Subsequently, however, in 1988, further changes saw the elimination in principle of all restrictions on private provision of medical care: already existing private practitioners were recognised, and full-time private entrepreneurship was legalised (Gaál 2004: 7). In addition, in the same year the financing of the health care system was transferred from taxation and direct government control to compulsory social insurance contributions under the Social Insurance Fund, which was detached from the central budget and became the main means of financing the operation of health institutions (Gaál 2004: 102). Of course, by the time of the regime change of 1989–90 there was little time for these changes to have much impact. However, it was in the context, and on the basis of the attempted reforms of the communist state-managed system that the further changes associated with post-communist transformation then took place.

The post-communist political framework

Hungary's political transition was elite-driven, negotiated and peaceful (Cox and Mason 1999; Gallai 2003). Uniquely in the region, an early pluralisation took place, and a multiparty system had already emerged before the first free elections (Bozóki 2003). Extensive modifications to the Constitution resulted in the creation of a political system comprising a single-chamber parliament and an indirectly elected president as head of state with relatively weak powers. The government was fully subordinated to parliament, but within parliament the requirement of a qualified two-thirds majority in a number of areas granted strong veto power to the political minority. Further institutional guarantees against the concentration of power included a complex system of checks and balances provided by the Constitutional Court, parliamentary commissioners and the State Audit Office (Körösényi et al. 2003). The new system enabled the free foundation and operation of political parties, business chambers, trade unions, interest groups and associations. However, while Hungarian society in the 1980s had been characterised by a significant growth of civic associations, and some interest groups had played an important role in events leading to the end of communist rule, in the post-communist political system both activists and resources gravitated to the political parties, resulting in the 'over-particisation' of Hungarian politics (Ágh 1998: 22).

Between 1990 and 2008, all Hungarian governments were formed as coalitions of parties and they mostly enjoyed majority support in parliament, enabling them to control the process of law-making (Körösényi et al. 2003). After the elections of 1998, increasing centralisation within the government, stronger coordination and leadership, a forceful personnel policy, and a new more hostile attitude towards the opposition all contributed to a change in the context of policy-making. As a result, the executive branch and its head, the prime minister, considerably strengthened their power vis-à-vis the other political institutions. That development was reinforced by changes in 2006 to the legal and political environment of the cabinet (Gallai and Lánczi 2006). As a result, the Hungarian political system began to shift from a mixed system towards a majority model (Lijphart 1992) at the same time as the transformation of the party system demonstrated a similar development by moving from 'moderate pluralism' (Sartori 1976) towards a quasi-two-party system.

Compared with other countries in the region, the Hungarian party system demonstrated a relatively high level of stability and consolidation (Bozóki 2003). While in the first three elections fluctuating voter choices made the political pendulum swing from side to side, after 1998 there was a concentration of support for the main two political parties. In 2002 and 2006 the Hungarian Socialist Party (MSZP) and Fidesz were each able to obtain more than 40 percent of the votes. The concentration of votes and the stabilisation of two main parties led to the emergence of a quasi-two-party system, which was characterised by bitter conflicts and deep antagonism.

The polarisation of politics became even more pronounced in 2006, when the (formerly unprecedented) re-election of the incumbent government was followed by austerity measures, the leaking of the infamous 'lies' speech by Prime Minister Gyurcsány, and the escalation of street riots followed by police brutality during the national holiday. The discredited prime minister subordinated governance to his own political survival (Gallai 2008), and after losing a referendum on symbolic reform measures in 2008,[4] he even sacrificed the coalition and, for the first time since 1990, a single-party, minority cabinet was formed. Although the cabinet survived several crucial votes in parliament, the implications of the international financial crisis forced the prime minister to step down. The new, temporary cabinet devoted its incomplete (one-year) term to crisis management and introduced some very unpopular cuts. Dissatisfaction with the government, increasing distrust in politics and politicians, and growing disappointment with the outcome of transition had shaken the Hungarian party system.[5] The parliamentary elections of 2010 produced a major defeat of the Socialist Party and a landslide victory for Fidesz. At the same time, two new, anti-establishment parties entered parliament: the radical nationalist Movement for a Better Hungary (Jobbik) and the alternative left green party – Politics Can Be Different (LMP).

Institutional and political changes in the Hungarian health sector after 1989

After the change of political regime, the institutional landscape of the health sector was altered considerably as part of a more extensive market-based transformation of the economy, and Hungary's increasing exposure to globalising influences. The roles of regulator, owner, purchaser and service provider were separated from one another (Gaál 2004: 12), and their relations were generally established by laws, decrees and contracts. In 1989, public institutions were deprived of their previously privileged position in the provision of medical care. The new law (Act 4/1989) declared that all natural persons and legal entities were allowed to pursue medical activities, and to set up and maintain health institutions, on condition that they met the appropriate conditions concerning personnel and professional standards (Gaál 2004: 28, 102). In principle this paved the way for the privatisation of health care, but the government of the time chose not to follow this with more specific legislation to establish rules and guidelines for privatisation or to stipulate what services could or could not be privatised.

In the new political system, the size and structure of the annual health budget were now to be determined by parliament, while the central government (the 'cabinet') would now be responsible for the formulation of policy concerning health and the financing of medical and public health services. The making of health policy became the responsibility of a specific ministry: between 1990 and 1998 this was the Ministry of Public Welfare, then after government reorganisation in 1998, the Ministry of Health.[6] For professional assistance on specific medical issues, the minister in charge of health could rely on several advisory bodies. The largest, the National Health Council, set up in 1999, brought together thirty representatives of professional chambers, trade unions, universities, scientific associations, patients' groups and local authorities to discuss the directions and key issues of health policy.

After 1989, governments at national level also attempted to foster a more reflexive approach to governance in relation to health care, and a range of mechanisms for consultation with stakeholders and interested policy actors was established. Health professionals established three chambers: the Hungarian Medical Chamber in 1989, the Hungarian Chamber of Pharmacists in 1994 and the Chamber of Professional Health Workers in 2003. The chambers issue codes of ethics for medical practice, and have the right to impose sanctions on those who do not comply. They also play an important role in professional training and further education, and have the right to be consulted on various medical issues; the Hungarian Medical Chamber has veto powers concerning the conditions of contracts between medical doctors and the National Health Insurance Administration. Between 1994 and 2007, membership of the chambers was made compulsory and the chambers were also assigned a regulatory role.[7] Other important professional organisations are the Alliance of Hospitals and the Association of Health Financial Managers, which tend to express similar views to each other on the issue of hospital financing.

After the regime change, numerous new trade unions were organised at local, sectoral and national level. In the health sector, the Democratic Trade Union of Health Workers became the largest union. While some professional bodies have tried to stay out of political issues, the leadership of both the trade union and the Hungarian Medical Chamber have often become involved in policy issues that have been divisive in terms of party politics. Union representatives also participate in various forums of interest reconciliation but, despite their loud voice, occasional demonstrations and strikes, their impact on policies has proved to be rather limited. The reputation of the unions in general, and in particular that of the main successor confederation – the National Confederation of Hungarian Trade Unions – suffered a heavy blow in 1997–98, when financial scandals surrounding the operation of the Health Insurance self-government (which consisted of union and employer representatives) were revealed in the press.

Patients' associations have mushroomed since the regime change. There are more than 100 registered patients' associations, most of which are usually organised along groups of illnesses and conditions.[8] While these represent specific patients' interests, other organisations focus on patients' rights with the aim of providing legal protection.[9] Representation as a collective right of patients has appeared only gradually, and its scope remained limited for many years (Molnár 2001; Heuer 2002). Nevertheless, patients' organisations have gained representation in advisory and coordinating bodies such as the National Health Council, regional health councils,[10] hospital supervisory councils,[11] county ethics committees,[12] and waiting list committees, and they also take part in pharmaceutical price negotiations. Moreover, they are free to register with parliament and the Ministry of Health to be incorporated into a system of compulsory consultations.[13] However, despite the emergence of these professional and interest-based organisations, and although health care reforms in the first few years of transformation resulted in more decentralised and less concentrated institutional arrangements, decisions on the financing of health policies and health services remained highly centralised.

The first main reform in the financing of the sector began in 1992, when social insurance contributions were divided into health and pension insurance contributions, and the Social Insurance Fund was split accordingly. The separation of the newly established Health Insurance Fund was accomplished a year later, when the administration of the health and pension funds was also divided into two, and the emerging National Health Insurance Administration became the single purchaser in the state-run health insurance system.

Members' contributions are the main source of revenues to the Health Insurance Fund. They account for around 70 percent of all revenues, while the rest of the revenues mostly come from the central budget. Health contributions are paid by both employers and employees. However, there are two social problems that curtail the size of the revenue:[14] first, the relatively small proportion of the economically active population who pay contributions – of Hungary's 10 million inhabitants, only 3.7 million pay contributions; second, relatively widespread tax evasion, with nearly half of all working employees reportedly only earning the minimum wage, while quite a few still work in the black and grey economies. Therefore reducing the incentives for and the possibilities of evading payment of contributions became a key objective of the government. In the mid-1990s, the contribution base was broadened and a new lump-sum, hypothecated tax was introduced, while the rate of health insurance contributions paid by employers was actually decreased. A few years later, the government decreased the rate of health insurance contributions further, while the hypothecated health tax was extended and increased. After 2006, more emphasis was laid on the criteria for eligibility to access services, but although that move increased the number of contribution-payers successfully, due to macroeconomic imbalances it was impossible to make further decreases to the level of contributions.

Of all expenditure, nearly 80 percent is devoted to payment of service providers, while around 17 percent is spent on cash benefits. The remaining 3 percent is mostly devoted to paying pension contributions for mothers on maternity leave. Of the cash benefits, more than three-quarters is allocated for financing the costs of maternity leave (36 percent) and sick leave (40 percent). Of in-kind benefits, the Fund spends more than 30 percent on subsidising medicines, 30 percent on buying services in active inpatient care, close to 10 percent on outpatient care, and around 9 percent on primary care – of which a quarter goes to finance dental services and three-quarters to general practitioners. The remaining 20 percent or so is allocated for the purchase of medical services such as chronic care, diagnostics, dialysis and ambulance services, as well as medical equipment.[15]

Within the new system, the detailed organisation of services and the operation of particular medical and health institutions were devolved from central government, mainly to local governments. When democratic local governments were established in 1990, they were granted very broad areas of competence, including infrastructure development, primary and secondary education, local social services and local health services. As a consequence of taking responsibility for health services, they gained ownership over most primary care facilities, hospitals and polyclinics. Since then, municipal governments have been free to decide how to organise and guarantee health provision at the local level. They may provide services using their own institutions and public employees, opt for contracting out particular services to private companies, or for full-scale privatisation of institutions or services. Several bigger municipalities own local hospitals and outpatient clinics, but other units of secondary care are typically subordinated to county governments.[16] The operational costs of providing services in both municipal and county institutions are paid from the Health Insurance Fund, while capital costs (investments, maintenance and development) are the responsibility of the local governments as owners, who have usually had to rely on additional financial support from the central governmental budget.

The reform of health policy has faced major challenges in the post-communist period, resulting from a mixture of demographic changes, the dismantling of the communist system of service provision and the development of a market economy, among a range of other connected changes in society and the economy. The initial reforms of the early 1990s took place in the context of the transitional recession that affected all the former communist countries, and thereafter the costs of health care have presented serious problems for successive governments. Within this general economic context, the attempt to shift the financing of health care from the central budget to a contribution-based insurance fund was never completely successful, and the government was faced with a continuing need for supplementary payments from the budget. These general problems exacerbated the problem of hospital financing (Kornai 2009). In addition, the establishment of democratic local governments was not accompanied by the setting up of a sound system of financing local services and, as a result, local governments remained chronically short of resources for funding the capital and running costs of hospitals and other health care institutions for which they had been given responsibility under the reforms.[17]

The remaining sections of this chapter focus on two of the major issues of health care policy that have confronted successive governments: the financing of health care and the regulation of privatisation.

Financing

For most of the past three decades, the Hungarian economy has been characterised by fiscal imbalances, external debt and slow economic growth.[18] As a result, persistent economic difficulties have forced successive Hungarian governments to introduce austerity programmes. In the early 1990s, existing structural problems inherited from the communist period were deepened by the transformation crisis. Economic needs and electoral considerations mostly translated into stop–go policy cycles. After the regime change, four serious fiscal adjustments programmes were implemented – in 1991, 1995, 2006 and 2009, respectively.[19] While all four programmes involved considerable cuts in public spending, the health sector was affected particularly severely in 1995 and 2006.[20]

In 1995, the health budget was cut so considerably that its funding hit the lowest point in its post-1990 history. The Health Insurance Fund stopped both the financing of dental services and the subsidising of spa treatments.[21] Co-payment, which had already existed in the case of paying for medicines, was also introduced for patient transport. Responsibility for health services at workplaces was transferred from the state to employers. Last, but not least, the number of hospital beds was reduced considerably. The austerity package provoked severe criticism that included legal objections. Several motions were submitted to the Constitutional Court, which ruled that some of the measures were in conflict with the Constitution and other standing laws. The Court also declared that standing regulations were violated by the way hospital capacities had been reduced.[22] The government accepted the criticism and opted for indirect intervention instead, when a year later a need-based formula, involving the number of hospital beds per county, was introduced and used for determining the necessary health care capacities. Since the formula demanded further cuts in most counties, the outcome was very much in line with the capacity-reduction of the previous year. This time, however, the actual means and dispersion of the reduction was left to the county assemblies. Although very few institutions were closed down, the overall reduction was roughly the same as in 1995 (around 9000 beds).

In this context, health expenditure in Hungary fell far below the average of the OECD countries. In 2007, Hungary's expenditure was $1388 (PPP), compared with the OECD average of $2984 (PPP). In the Višegrad region, health spending was the highest in the Czech Republic at $1626 (PPP), while

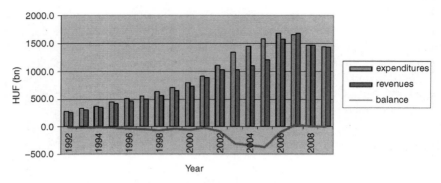

Figure 7.1 The balance of the Health Insurance Fund
Source: data provided by the Health Insurance Fund, www.oep.hu

the lowest was in Poland at $1035 (PPP), with Hungary and Slovakia falling somewhere in between.[23] Moreover, as can be seen in Figure 7.1, for most years between 1992 and 2009 the Health Insurance Fund was running with a significant deficit. Although each of the twenty sub-budgets was meant to operate within an upper ceiling, and service financing had also included mechanisms to protect caps on expenditure, after 2002 the balance of the Fund started to deteriorate dramatically.

In response to the growing crisis situation in 2006, after the parliamentary elections of that year the returning Socialist–Free Democrat government introduced major changes in the financing of the sector. First, the minister for health readjusted the cap on financing by setting it at 95 percent of the formerly reported activities (Sinkó 2008). Expenditures were reduced by merging some hospitals and closing down others; restraining the performance of inpatient service providers; regulating the prescribing of medicines; forcing pharmaceutical companies to compete and to contribute to the HIF; and cutting other medical spending. At the same time, the government decided to reduce hospital capacities. Hospitals were classified by range of services. Some were allowed to provide the widest range of health services, whilst others were given lower classifications (Mihályi and Molnár 2006). The highest category was reserved for clinics and hospitals of regional importance, while the lowest category comprised small local hospitals with rather limited capacities, resources and activities.

The outcome was a considerable cut. Five hospitals were closed down, eleven were transformed into chronic care rehabilitation centres, six hospitals were merged into one with reduced capacities, and active inpatient care capacity was reduced by 26 percent, that is, by 15,500 beds, of which around 7000 were transferred to chronic care, resulting in a 35 percent increase there. In the original versions of the cuts package, the key criteria for deciding on hospital closures were redundant capacity, shortages of professionals and whether the institution made a loss. However, as a result of political lobbying, the final list of affected institutions was distorted, and this undermined the legitimacy of the arguments.

At the same time as making these cuts, revenues to the HIF were to be increased by the introduction of co-payment in both primary care and active inpatient care, and by a stricter monitoring of eligibility for health services that brought in many new contributors to the HIF. From 2007, the government introduced the so-called visiting fee and hospital fee. The former had to be paid by patients to their doctor after each visit.[24] The latter was paid by patients to the hospital they had stayed in. The fees were set at HUF 300 (about €1.1 at the time) per visit and per day, respectively.

The overall result of the changes was very positive in financial terms. For the first time in its history, the balance of the HIF showed a surplus, even though the sector – even in nominal terms – had lost substantial resources (revenues) to the central budget. However, in social terms the changes had some very negative consequences. In order to successfully eliminate the Fund deficit, the government applied existing administrative and financial brakes on health expenditures with no regard to their medical and political consequences. The government did not take account of cancelled surgeries, expanding waiting lists, more expensive medicines, criticism of co-payments, and opposition to the closure of institutions. Although the co-payment fees were relatively modest, they were very unpopular and became the target of a bitter political conflict between the governing MSZP and the senior opposition party, Fidesz. Moreover, since most decisions were imposed on the sector (Dózsa 2008), the government was unable to win the support of the affected interest organisations.

The widespread opposition to the changes was reflected politically in the referendum of March 2008, in which a question on co-payments became one of the main symbolic issues. The referendum was the result of a strong opposition initiative to block government policies and create tension within the coalition. It was initiated by Fidesz on 23 October 2006, and consisted of three questions. These referred to hospital attendance fees, fees for visits to doctors, and also to whether students in higher education should pay tuition fees. The outcome was a strong protest vote against the government, and both co-payment fees and tuition fees were rejected with a convincing majority. The results, with a turnout of over 50 percent, higher than opinion polls had expected, showed that there were clear majorities in favour of abolishing all the fees. As far as the two questions relating to health policy were concerned, the results were 84.08 percent against hospital fees, and 82.42 percent against doctors' consultation fees.

Privatisation of health institutions and services

As noted above, general legislative and constitutional changes in the late 1980s made privatisation possible in principle, but no general policy on health care privatisation was developed by the national government. The major elements of privatisation that did take place on a national level were in 1992, when measures were introduced to enable family doctors' practices to become private businesses, and in 1994, when pharmacies were privatised. As a result, by the mid-1990s virtually all pharmacies had been privatised and 90 percent of family doctors were self-employed and working in private businesses.[25] However, the conservative coalition government of that period, led by the Hungarian Democratic Forum, did not seek to extend privatisation any further. Nevertheless, in reaction to the general shortage of health care funding and the problems of financing the operation of hospitals, the privatisation of health care provision, in the form of either the privatisation of particular services or the full-scale privatisation of hospitals, was a serious policy option at national and local levels, which soon appeared on the policy agenda. Thus the privatisation of some medical services and some institutions began to take place in a piecemeal and often unregulated fashion. From 1994 onwards, local governments in need of investment capital started to launch a series of privatisation deals that affected medical centres, clinics, and hospitals or hospital units. As a result, private enterprises became important contributors to laboratories, imaging diagnostics and other high-tech services. In many institutions, supplementary services such as washing, cleaning and maintenance were also contracted out to private enterprises. By the mid-1990s, nearly 90 percent of artificial kidney centres were run by private companies, and altogether around 10 percent of health services were provided by the private sector.

However, while privatisation was legally possible, and had become prevalent in some areas of medical services, the actual terms and conditions under which it took place remained unregulated. Local governments, the owners of most institutions, were free in principle to sell their property. The local government act had 'only' made them responsible for organising the provision of health services, while the ways and means for doing this had been left open for them to consider. At the same time, there was no effective legal environment for regulating the expanding private enterprises in the health sector. It was even the case that legislation introduced in relation to other issues had the effect of limiting the extent of possible privatisations. As late as 2002, just before the attempted introduction of specific legislation on health care privatisation, the scope for hospital privatisation was limited by the introduction of modifications to an act on targeted and earmarked subsidies to local governments. One of its provisions imposed a ten-year ban on the privatisation of those local government-owned health institutions that had received such subsidies any time after 1993. The ban was applied to roughly half of the county and larger municipal hospitals.

By the late 1990s, in this rather confusing and complex legal context, a debate was well under way on how the situation should be rationalised, how privatisation should take place in the sector, and the extent to which it should be permitted. The debate reflected divisions among ministries within government, as well as among different groups of medical professionals and other interest groups. On one hand, representatives of the Ministry of Welfare (later the Ministry of Health) and the National Health Insurance Fund favoured a predominantly publicly financed system in which particular services would be provided by enterprises of different ownership forms, including private, non-profit, local government-owned and state-owned. With only a few well defined exceptions, services were to be practically free of charge for patients, and private funds would be used only to operate supplementary schemes. On the other hand, the main concern of monetarist economists and Ministry of Finance representatives was to find a way considerably to reduce expenditures on public health. In their view, the exclusive use of public funds should be limited to a very small range of basic services and to the poorest sections of society. All other services should be paid for partly by patients, and private insurance schemes should be introduced. Obviously, private insurance companies gave strong backing to such ideas. There were also divisions between the main political parties, as will be discussed below, with the Socialists favouring more extensive privatisation than Fidesz. Among hospital directors and management members, the concept of managerial ownership gained the highest support. Other managers, many employees and unions considered physician ownership to be the most reasonable solution. However, some incumbent senior managers of institutions and senior medical professors and researchers tended to reject any changes at all to the ownership of hospitals.[26] A further question under debate was whether to privatise entire hospitals or only separate units providing particular services.

Attempts to regulate hospital privatisation

In the early 2000s, there were two attempts to regulate hospital privatisation: firstly in 2002 during the final months of the first Fidesz-led government of Viktor Orbán; and secondly in 2003, in the first year of the newly elected socialist-led government of Péter Medgyessy. Both aimed to facilitate financing and make the raising of private capital easier. In the end, however, both pieces of legislation were repealed, and privatisation in health care remained, by and large, an unregulated area.

The 'Mikola Act'

The act of 2002 was named after then health minister István Mikola of Fidesz. The Mikola Act addressed two issues: the problem of financing hospitals, and the status of health care employees. In keeping with Fidesz's general reservations concerning privatisation and neoliberal approaches to economic reform, their proposed legislation envisaged the partial or complete transfer of ownership of hospitals to public benefit associations or public foundations, and ruled out privatisation by for-profit companies or by physicians or pharmacists. The bill also introduced a change in the legal status of general practitioners. It reinforced their freelance status by awarding them ownership of their practices.[27] According to the minister, the proposed changes clarified privatisation options that were already possible under existing law, therefore the new legislation was only aimed at reinforcing and regulating already existing possibilities.

In the ensuing debate, the bill was criticised by outright opponents because it would restrict the range of non-state owners of hospitals and exclude for-profit owners, and by others because it would enable the sale of the most profitable units of health care institutions while leaving the economically weak and failing units in public ownership and in a potentially uncertain situation. Among the health professional groups, while the Hungarian Hospital Association, representing hospital directors, declined to express a view, arguing that hospital privatisation was a topic of a political nature and not a health professional issue, most other professional interest organisations, including the Democratic Trade Union of Medical Workers (EDDSZ) and the Hungarian Medical Chamber (MOK), rejected the proposal because they strongly opposed the possibility of what they saw as 'cherry picking', meaning the detachment and the sale of profitable units while leaving the economically depressed larger units to the state or local government.[28] Allowing subcontracting service providers to contract the National Health Fund directly was another heavily criticised provision in the text. Among business actors, however, the proposal attracted the support of one of the two dominant groups already operating in the health care sector, the Dutch-owned Euro-Medic and its sister companies. They invested mostly in very expensive computer diagnostic equipment, and favoured a range of options, from subcontracting for the operation of certain hospital units to the purchase of entire institutions.[29]

The bill also attracted considerable opposition in parliament, and initially it was rejected by parliament's standing committee on health affairs when the opposition members and Mánya Kristóf, a Fidesz MP, voted against it. However, Fidesz's parliamentary group came to the support of the bill and saw it through later stages of debate. The bill was passed by a vote of the majority governing coalition MPs, who ignored criticism from both within and outside parliament. The opposition parties (MSZP and the Alliance of Free Democrats – SZDSZ) argued that the implementation of the Mikola Act would lead to particularly serious problems in the areas of laboratory diagnosis and artificial kidney therapies, and they voted against the new law. The Act came into effect in March 2002, but the most disputed provisions were to come into force in 2003 and 2004. However, before the Act could be fully implemented, the parliamentary elections of 2002 produced a victory for the MSZP and consequently a change of government. The new health minister in the new MSZP–SZDSZ coalition government, Judit Csehák, initiated the suspension of those provisions of the Mikola Act that were already in force and announced that she would introduce new legislation on the financing and privatisation of service provision.

The 'Hospital Act' of 2003

The Mikola Act was repealed and replaced in 2003 by the so-called Hospital Act.[30] The new legislation, in contrast to the Mikola Act, and reflecting the more neoliberal approach of the coalition partners, aimed to generate private investment in the health sector and allow privatisation without any restrictions on either the sector or the for-profit nature of the investors. It thus permitted the privatisation of both the services and the real estate of health care institutions by for-profit investors. At the same time, also in contrast to the previous legislation, it excluded the privatisation of separate hospital or other health care institution units and thus avoided the problem perceived by critics of the Mikola Act of cherry picking profitable parts of a larger institution.[31]

The new legislation was particularly significant for the government, not only as a means of regulating the piecemeal privatisations that had been taking place, but also as a way of resolving the growing problems of financing health care: the government expected the Act to generate private investments in the health care sector, resulting in a higher level of service provision. Mainly for this reason, the new law avoided restrictions on the sector or the form of investors, and did not impose any ban on investors coming from the sector, or on enterprises of a for-profit nature. However, privatisation was to be conditional on the investors contributing to the institution's property by increasing the capital of the institution, and on the limitation of the stake acquired by investors to no more than 49 percent.

The new proposed legislation prompted a great deal of debate and provoked even more controversy than its predecessor. It was opposed by a wide range of different opinions, including the opposition parties (Fidesz and the Hungarian Democratic Forum – MDF), two extra-parliamentary parties, the Workers' Party and the Hungarian Justice and Life Party (MIÉP), and some civic circles and organisations representing patients' rights.[32] The Democratic Trade Union of Medical Workers (EDDSZ) rejected the entire bill, targeting its criticism mostly at the provision that allowed privatisation by for-profit enterprises. In their view, the bill had been designed only to serve the profits of investors. Moreover, a further demand of the EDDSZ leadership was the inclusion of health care legislation in the category of laws requiring a qualified two-thirds majority in parliament, a demand that was subsequently ignored by the government. On the other hand, the bill found strong support from the second of the two dominant business groups in health care, Prodia and its sister companies including Hospinvest, which had been established by Hungarian investors, initially in the field of less expensive laboratory diagnostics.[33] Following the publication of the bill, they declared an aim to establish and run a network of nine to twelve hospitals by obtaining their operation rights.[34]

Some organisations, including professional civil organisations such as the Hungarian Hospital Association, once again stayed out of the debate, while others again put forward a range of different criticisms, but sought to persuade the government to incorporate amendments rather than mounting outright opposition. The Hungarian Medical Chamber was split over the issue.[35] MOK president Péter Kupcsulik took part in direct talks with Prime Minister Péter Medgyessy, who promised to modify the bill in line with the expectations of Chamber leaders. The demands that were accepted included veto powers for hospital management in certain areas; priority to be given to doctors in privatisation; and favourable loans and state guarantee for doctors to take part in the privatisation. On the other hand, there was disagreement between MOK and the government on who should be included in the category of potential buyers, since the Chamber continued to reject the possibility of for-profit companies and producers of pharmaceuticals and other medical products becoming hospital owners. Although a compromise position was agreed between the government and the MOK leadership,[36] for a vocal section of MOK members the agreement was an unacceptable compromise, and they succeeded in bringing about a motion of no confidence in the MOK leadership. A new leadership was elected on 16 August 2003, Péter Kupcsulik was replaced as president by István Éger, and MOK then adopted the position that the government should withdraw the bill.

Despite the changing views within MOK, some of their original proposals found their way into the final version of the legislation, as did some amendments proposed by the Alliance of Social Professionals (3SZ).[37] Leading members of the Alliance, Zsuzsa Ferge, Éva Orosz and Kinga Göncz, met Health Minister Csehák as well as other ministers and members of parliament, and managed to gain support for some modifications to the bill, most notably the inclusion of a provision codifying the right of the state to buy back health institutions from private owners in the event of their bankruptcy.[38]

Furthermore, in response to criticism from existing for-profit hospital owners, a further amendment proposed that potential buyers would be required to present certain guarantees, and gain approval from the National Public Health Medical Officer Service and from the respective regional branch of the Hungarian Medical Chamber, as well as consulting with the trade unions that would be affected. These modifications were criticised, however, in that they would lead to the establishment of an over-regulated system.[39] In order to meet the conditions for privatisation, prospective buyers would have been subjected to a long process to collect all the necessary permits and opinions, and even then it was not at all certain permission would be granted.

Despite modifications to the bill, the opposition political parties maintained their more fundamentally negative views regarding the proposed legislation. The largest opposition party in parliament, Fidesz, vehemently rejected the idea of privatisation by for-profit companies. Their representatives described the proposal as a means of selling off public real estate properties in the health sector, and warned that certain business interests would be interested in buying hospitals only for their extremely valuable sites.[40] Some Fidesz MPs even claimed that the government had deliberately pushed hospitals to the brink of bankruptcy in order to appoint a commissioner, István Győrfi, in charge of consolidation,[41] and to justify the need for privatisation. The other parliamentary opposition party, the Hungarian Democratic Forum, supported the basic idea of privatisation, but opposed the proposed conditions entailed in the legislation. Both of the two main extra-parliamentary parties, the Workers' Party and MIÉP, respectively of the far-left and the far-right, expressed their basic opposition to private capital taking over hospitals.

The amended bill was approved by parliament on 16 June despite the level of opposition. The MPs of the governing MSZP–SZDSZ coalition voted for the bill,[42] while the opposition Fidesz and MDF representatives were against. However, such was their depth of opposition to the idea of selling hospitals as public property that the opposition parties continued their attacks on the new law even after it was passed. Their first step was to call on the President of the Republic to exercise his legal veto, to refuse to sign the bill, and to send it to the Constitutional Court for adjudication. The President consulted both the incumbent health minister and her predecessor, and decided to put a political veto on the Act. This meant that, instead of forwarding it to the Constitutional Court, which would have followed from a legal veto, he sent it back to parliament for reconsideration. The President argued that allowing for-profit companies to take over inpatient services from public providers would undermine equal access to high-level services. In his view, it was also worrying that companies trading with or producing medicines and medical equipment might also take a share in hospital privatisation, with the possible consequence that they could even become both seller and buyer of the same products. In his opinion, such a development would certainly limit competition and lead to higher prices. Moreover, he also criticised the government's failure to make public the findings of background studies of the possible implications of the Act.

However, the government remained intransigent. On 23 June, the same day as the President's veto was submitted to parliament, the MPs were called into an extraordinary session to debate it. The governing majority decided to override the presidential veto, which did not require a qualified two-thirds majority in parliament, and so the bill was approved once again. Before the vote, the opposition MPs left the chamber in protest against both the attitude of the governing majority and the absence of the prime minister, who had already gone on holiday. The second approval by parliament obliged the President to inaugurate the law. He did so, but he also turned to the Constitutional Court for clarification of the constitution. He asked for a decision on whether such a hurriedly organised and held debate, and the subsequent approval of the identical text, fulfilled the category of 'reconsideration'. He also asked for clarification of the conditions of his participation in the debate, since he had only received the agenda two days before the extraordinary session, less than required by the regulations.

The opposition parties also turned to the Constitutional Court. Fidesz challenged four elements of the Hospital Act and the way it had been adopted. The party argued that the Act would undermine the principle of equal access to health services, and would also make health sector employees vulnerable in case of takeovers by for-profit companies. In addition, they regarded privatisation as involving the potential loss of valuable state property, and argued that the legal environment would be uncertain after the adoption of the Act. They also criticised the lack of background and feasibility studies since the government was obliged by law to prepare such studies before submitting a bill to parliament. Finally, Fidesz stated that the way the Act was approved in the second round (the extra-ordinary session) was against the Constitution, and also violated the rules of parliamentary procedure because the MPs had not received the agenda in sufficient time according to the rules. The MDF also submitted its legal reservations to the Constitutional Court. Besides challenging the way the extraordinary session was held, the party protested against provisions in the Act dealing with the role of churches, and against the possibility of for-profit and intra-sectoral pharmaceutical companies taking over health institutions.

While the opposition attempted to block the legislation, the Act came into force in mid-July 2003, and was followed by subsequent government decrees that elaborated the actual forms and conditions of contracting for service provision. However, in December 2003 the Constitutional Court ruled that parliament had violated the Constitution when it failed to discuss the President's arguments. Therefore, without examining the contents of the Act, the Court declared that the procedure of the adoption of the Act was unconstitutional, and the Hospital Act was therefore null and void. The governing majority could have responded to the Court ruling by adopting the same, or a modified, version of the text in a constitutionally correct way, but they chose not to take this course because of other developments that had been taking place in parallel.

In July 2003, at the time of the adoption of the Act, the extra-parliamentary Workers' Party had announced a call for a national referendum on hospital privatisation, to prevent the 'separation of hospitals for the rich and for the poor'. The question to be voted on was as follows: 'Do you agree that public health institutions, hospitals, shall remain the property of the state and local governments, and that parliament shall therefore repeal the law which is inconsistent with that?' In August and November 2003, the National Election Committee and the Constitutional Court, respectively, issued their consent to the referendum initiative. Fidesz announced its support of the initiative and joined in the process of collecting signatures in support. When the Constitutional Court's decision that the Hospital Act was null and void was announced, the referendum organisers decided to continue collecting signatures calling for a referendum in order to prevent the government pushing a similar bill through parliament. The collection and verification of more than 200,000 supporting signatures obliged parliament to call a referendum on the initiative.

The referendum, which was held in December 2004, contained two questions. One was on the privatisation of health institutions, the other on the question of dual citizenship for Hungarians abroad. According to the regulations of the time, for a referendum vote to be successful, more than half of the valid votes cast, representing more than a quarter of all eligible voters, had to give the same answer of 'yes' or 'no' to the questions posed. In the 2004 referendum, the votes cast for both questions fell short of these requirements. In the case of the privatisation issue, nearly 3 million people, only 37 percent of all eligible voters, cast their votes. 'Yes' votes were cast by 65 percent of all those who voted (but this was only 23.89 percent of all voters), while 'No' received the support of 35 percent of the votes cast (but only 12.58 percent of all voters). However, although the referendum fell short of imposing a legally binding ban on hospital privatisation, the outcome gave the government a political lesson that had policy implications. The very clear majority against hospital privatisation, which was highlighted by the much more closely split vote on dual citizenship,[43] suggested that a considerable proportion of government supporters agreed with the opposition on this issue, and it would be politically dangerous to pursue further the idea of hospital privatisation. It was probably mainly for this reason that the government decided to refrain from any further revision and resubmission of the Hospital Act.

Despite the failure of the two legislative attempts at establishing a regulated approach to hospital privatisation, the privatisation of health institutions and health services did not stop, while the transformation of public institutions into 'non-profit corporations' had also begun. Following the failure of the referendum attempt to ban privatisation legally, nothing hampered these processes, although their scope and scale remained limited. In the hope of future benefits, two main groups invested in the sector. One of these, however, reported bankruptcy in 2009.[44] In recent years, unfavourable financial conditions and the lack of respective regulations have hampered the raising of private capital for the sector. Moreover, public sentiment remains sceptical about private enterprises in the health sector,[45] and medical staff have also been alienated by a number of scandals concerning hospitals under private management.[46]

Conclusion: policy problems and failures

The attempts of successive governments to regulate hospital privatisation resulted in the failure of two pieces of legislation and an invalid referendum against privatisation, which nevertheless showed a convincing majority of voters against the privatisation of hospitals, the lack of proper regulation, and the expression of strong public sentiments against private investors. The two pieces of legislation discussed above involved intensive preparation and deliberation, and extensive debates over the policy issues between govern-ments, competing political parties and a range of other interested policy actors. However, the basic issues that prompted the attempts at legislation were not resolved. While one piece of legislation was passed by one government, it was quickly rescinded by the next. The general impression was therefore of policy drift while the underlying problems continued to accumulate.

One criticism of both pieces of legislation has been that they were piecemeal and too narrowly focused on particular aspects of the problems, to the exclusion of other issues. In a report on functional privatisation, the State Audit Office concluded that the sector was lacking a strategy that could determine – in line with health policy objectives – the possible size, role and investment areas of private capital (Állami 2009: 17). However, in order to explain the situation more fully, it is necessary to examine key aspects of the character of the policy process in Hungarian politics, of which the specific case of health care policy is one example. Major factors in this respect have been the character of the relations between different policy actors, the predominance of the prime minister and the national government in policy-making, the predominance of political parties over other policy actors, and the increasingly bitter ideological and policy division between the two main political parties that have formed successive governments in Hungary (Gallai 2009).

Relations between policy actors and impediments to effective interest representation

The relationship between government and civil society in the achievement of effective governance in health policy-making, and hospital privatisation in particular, has been complex and problematic. On one hand, a range of institutional mechanisms have helped to facilitate dialogue and consultation, including free registration of groups with parliament and ministries, a system of consultations, and representation on various advisory and coordinating bodies. The story of the legislation on hospital privatisation offers several examples of the influence of various social actors in the formulation and drafting of the legislation, such as the proposals of 3SZ and MOK relating to the Hospital Act of 2003, discussed above. It can also be noted that market actors usually enjoy greater potential in representing interests and have more impact on legislation and decision-making. For example, in regard to the hospital acts, drafts were drawn up in line with the interests of particular investors, although these were watered down at the parliamentary stage or modified by medical professional interests also channelled in at that stage.

On the other hand, our examples also showed that in the health sector, the influence of social groups strongly depends on the will of the governing forces, which makes interest representation over-politicised. Their opinion is usually requested at short notice and is only occasionally taken into account. The lack of significant policy influence is explained partly by financial and operational shortcomings, since their organisation is usually weak and the extent of their expertise is often limited. Fragmentation, strong political differences and personal conflicts also impede interest representation. Our examples indicate that the structure of interest representation is fragmented. There are several players, with low membership and credibility problems, and they each focused separately on different issues so that, at best, they achieved minor amendments on specific points in the legislation. It is generally true that associations and interest groups often lack the necessary resources and personnel to engage in detailed consultation or effective lobbying. Most groups did not have enough expertise to influence decision-making effectively. The centralisation of decision-making and the increasing dominance of government had further serious consequences for the effectiveness of interest groups. In a situation where most interest groups have limited personnel and financial resources, they are often strongly dependent on government and political parties, leading to a situation of over-politicised interest representation. As noted above in the case of business groups, most influence is achieved when interest groups are supported by political actors.

The influence of social actors has been strongest when their interests have coincided with those of opposition political actors and they have been able to block reform initiatives at design or implementation stages. In these cases, the social actors, although they often lack professional capacities, have represented strong incumbent interests against restructuring, have been able to refer to public sentiment and have made use of referendum opportunities. Our clearest example in the area of health policy is where the medical elite – individually and through organised interest groups and companies – have lobbied against transparent financing, against reforms and against further financial burdens.

The role of government and electoral competition

The role of government itself in the wider process of governance is also important. Ironically, as government became increasingly centralised under the strong guidance of the Office of the Prime Minister, and as the role of government officials became increasingly politicised, centralised governments began to pay more attention to electoral politics and the bipartisan race with the opposition than to issues of effective governance. While this began under Orbán's first government between 1998 and 2002, it became a predominant characteristic under Gyurcsány, who succeeded in creating a situation where the conditions of exercising power gained priority over the objectives of governance (Gallai 2008). This acted as an impediment to the introduction of major reforms that ran the risk of making the government unpopular. Indeed, government options for reform and for introducing significant reforms came most easily at times of serious crisis situations, as for example with the introduction of the Bokros package of 1995, or the Bajnai package in the summer of 2009. In other circumstances, taking a strong initiative or the use of bureaucratic control was more usually subject to careful balancing between electoral considerations and financial sustainability. In the case of the legislation on hospital privatisation, such factors can be observed affecting the introduction of both acts.

The historical/ideological cleavage and party/electoral politics

Although the main cleavage described above between the MSZP and Fidesz has historical roots, since the Socialists are the post-communist successor party and Fidesz has emerged as the largest force rooted in the non-communist opposition of the late 1980s, the bitterness of the division has increased in recent years. Initially there was cooperation between rival politicians in some policy areas, for example the consensus on social insurance reform guidelines in 1991, and close cooperation among MPs and policy experts.[47] However, in examining health care policy, we have noted that the trend towards the concentration of the party system, and the emergence of a quasi-bipartisan structure, has been accompanied by strong polarisation over the policy issues, including examples of the total opposition to government measures by non-government MPs. This has resulted in U-turns in policies, especially following a change of government after elections, and most notably in the successive acts on hospital privatisation, the expulsion of undisciplined party members,[48] and the use of referenda by the opposition to block government initiatives.

Thus, while at one level the problems of achieving effective policy-making in the area of health care in Hungary can be examined as a narrative of the events and contestations of democratic politics, a deeper understanding can be achieved if these events are located within an analysis of the key features of the contemporary Hungarian political system that has emerged in the years since the end of communist rule. These include the increasing dominance of political parties combined with a weak influence from grassroots civil society and an increasing cleavage between what have become the two main parties in an increasingly two-party system. The predominance of parties over social actors, and the increasingly bitter division between the two main parties, have contributed to the weakness of other policy actors and their dependence on alliances with political parties to have an effective voice. The elite-based character of the consensual transition of power that took place in 1989–90 has left much unfinished business between the successors of communist rule in the Socialist Party and the successors of the opposition in Fidesz, and the dominance of these parties and the bitter divisions between them have created barren ground for the role of social actors more widely and the development of effective governance.

Notes

1 The research on which this chapter is based was funded in the UK by a Leverhulme Trust Research Fellowship (RF/7/RFG/2004/0349) for Terry Cox, and in Hungary

by a grant from the New Széchenyi Plan (TÁMOP-4.1.1.A-10/2/KMR-2010-0011) for Sándor Gallai.

2 That policy line made the Minister of Health one of the least popular politicians in Hungary, and the surrounding political conflicts forced him to resign.

3 Interview with Éva Kereszty, 10 March 2006.

4 These included two health policy issues, as discussed below.

5 According to a survey by Pew Research Center, Hungarians are the least satisfied with the outcome of transition (Pew Research 2009).

6 Most recently, after the elections of 2010, the Ministry of Health has been merged into the newly created Ministry of National Resources.

7 In 2007, however, in retaliation for their political opposition to the Minister for Health, compulsory membership was eliminated and their regulatory role was curtailed. That policy was reversed once again with the change in government as the current cabinet decided to restore the institution of compulsory membership.

8 In practice, however, several organisations have very small active leaderships. In their cases, media appearances tend to be more important than attempts to consult with government on prospective legislation. Interview with Éva Kereszty, 10 March 2006.

9 Interview with Judit Csehák, 27 March 2006.

10 Regional health councils were founded in each of the seven administrative regions of the country in 2005. They monitor and assess regional health programmes, give advice on the allocation of regional capacities and conciliate between the interests of regional stakeholders.

11 In 1999, supervisory councils were set up in hospitals to monitor their operation, give opinions and make proposals to institution managements.

12 In 1999, local ethics committees were set up in every health institution to issue protocols on ethical questions and make general recommendations. Individual cases, on the other hand, were originally investigated in the respective committees of the Hungarian Medical Chamber, but in 2007 that competence was transferred to the newly established county ethics committees.

13 The ministries are obliged to consult interest organisations of social groups on draft proposals. Organisations have to register with a particular ministry, then they automatically receive draft proposals on which they may give an opinion. When registered with parliament, they can receive draft bills for comment, but they may only attend the meetings of the respective standing committees by invitation. Interview with Éva Kereszty, 10 March 2006.

14 Interview with László Skultéty, 29 March 2005.

15 Own calculations from the data of the 2009 balance of the Fund. www.oep.hu/pls/portal/docs/PAGE/LAKOSSAG/OEPHULAK_UVEGZSEB/KOLTSEGVETESEK/P%C3%89NZFORGALMI_2010_J%C3%9ALIUS.pdf

16 That arrangement will most likely change, and the central government and its county representatives will acquire control over most institutions under a new act on local government that is in preparation at the time of writing.

17 Interview with László Skultéty, 29 March 2005.

18 The only marked exception was the period 1997–2003.

19 They went under the names of the Kupa, Bokros, Gyurcsány and Bajnai programmes, respectively. The former two were named after the incumbent finance ministers during those years, while the latter two were named after the prime ministers then in power.

20 A recent readjustment plan (named after a successful nineteenth-century finance minister, Kálmán Széll) also envisages a considerable outflow from the health budget to the central budget.

21 A year later, tooth-preservation treatments were once again added to the list of publicly funded services.

22 The Minister for Welfare had instructed the National Health Insurance Administration on how much capacity to contract for with individual service providers.
23 OECD Health Data 2009, www.oecd.org/health/healthdata
24 While this meant an extra revenue for the general practitioners, their overall situation hardly improved as the government also decided to cut back resources available for them to purchase new equipment.
25 The typical exceptions were some hospital pharmacies, and young doctors who were hired by the National Institute for Primary Health Care (OALI) to work in remote villages that were not sufficiently attractive to private practitioners.
26 Interview with Eszter Sinkó, 7 March 2006.
27 This meant that a retiring GP could supplement his/her pension by selling his/her practice to a new doctor, who would take over the retiring doctor's patients.
28 Interview with Géza Gyenes, 20 February 2006.
29 Interview with anonymous health expert, 2005.
30 The status of health employees, which had also been the subject of the Mikola Act, was settled later in a separate bill.
31 Interview with Mihály Kökény, 7 March 2006.
32 Interview with Éva Kereszty, 10 March 2006.
33 Interview with anonymous health expert, 2006.
34 Their efforts were reportedly supported by Socialist MP Mihály Kökény, who served as political state secretary under Csehák and succeeded her as Minister for Health when she decided to step down. Interview with health expert, 2005.
35 Interview with László Skultéty, 29 March 2005.
36 Interview with Géza Gyenes, 20 March 2006.
37 3SZ comes from the acronym Szociális Szakmai Szövetség.
38 Interview with Éva Kereszty, 10 March 2006.
39 Interview with László Skultéty, 29 March 2005.
40 Interview with Árpád Gógl, 6 March 2006.
41 The commissioner hired experts from the private company Perfect, owned by Altus, the flagship enterprise of Ferenc Gyurcsány, who at the time served as aide to Prime Minister Medgyess. Interview with anonymous health expert, 2005.
42 Despite the administrative hurdles, the liberal SZDSZ also voted for the bill, although it favoured a large-scale privatisation that would also cover the National Health Insurance system.
43 51.6 percent voted in favour, while 48.4 percent were against. (For exact figures and details see www.valasztas.hu/nepszav04/main_hu.html)
44 See www.heol.hu/heves/kozelet/hospinvest-felszamolas-heves-megye-nem-vallalja-az-adossagot-244566
45 See for example www.virtus.hu/?id=detailed_article&aid=22336
46 A corresponding report by the State Audit Office offers a comprehensive overview and assessment of the contribution of private enterprises to the operation of hospitals (Állami 2009).
47 See for example Gallai (1999).
48 A few local representatives of Fidesz were expelled from the party because they did not share the official (critical) policy line on hospital privatisation. See for example www.figyelo.hu/belfold/20080707/kizartak_fideszbol_korhazprivatizalokat

References

Ágh, A. (1998) The Politics of Central Europe, London: Sage.
Állami, S. (2009) Jelentés az egyes kórházi tevékenységek kiszervezésének ellenőrzéséről, No. 0921, 2009. www.asz.hu/ASZ/jeltar.nsf/0/41F5B0BD0EB6BBAEC1257603004C30B3/$File/0921J000.pdf

Bozóki, A. (2003) *Politikai pluralizmus Magyaroszágon, 1987–2002*, Századvég Kiadó.

Cox, T. and Mason, B. (1999) *Social and Economic Transformation in East Central Europe*, Cheltenham, UK: Edward Elgar.

Dózsa, C. (2008) '2006–2007-es évek az egészségügyben: reformtervek és programok kavalkádja', in S. Péter and L. Vass (eds), *Magyarország politikai évkönyve 2007-ről*. II. kötet, Budapest: Demokrácia Kutatások Magyar Központja Közhasznú Alapítvány.

Gaál, P. (2004) *Health Care Systems in Transition: Hungary*, Copenhagen: WHO Regional Office for Europe on behalf of the European Observatory on Health Systems and Policies.

Gallai, S. (1999) 'A nyugdíjreform: kényszerk és kételyek', in *Parlamenti pártok és törvényhozás 1997–1998*, MAPI-kötetek No. 2, Budapest.

——(2003) 'Politikai rendszerváltás Magyarországon', in S. Gallai and G. Török (eds), *Politika és politikatudomány*, Budapest: Aula Kiadó.

——(2008) 'Kormányzás és hatalom: a kreativitás tétje', in P. Balogh, B. Dobos, B. Nagy and A. Szűcs (eds), *60 éves a Közgazdaságtudományi Egyetem: A Jubileumi Tudományos Konferencia alkalmából készült tanulmányok*, Társadalomtudományi Kar, IV, Budapest: Aula.

——(2009) 'Hungary: a democratic polity under challenge', in T. Buksiński (ed.), *Democracy in Western and Post-Communist Countries*, Frankfurt am Main: Peter Lang.

Gallai, S. and Lánczi, T. (2006) 'Személyre szabott kormányzás – A második Gyurcsány-kormány anatómiája', in G. Karácsony (ed.), *Parlamenti választás 2006*; DKMKA–BCE Politikatudományi Intézet.

Heuer, O. (ed.) (2002) *Betegjogok Magyarországon – Szabályok és gyakorlat*, Budapest: Társaság a Szabadságjogokért.

Kornai, J. (2009) 'The soft budget constraint syndrome in the hospital sector', *Society and Economy*, 31: 5–31.

Körösényi, A., Tóth, C. and Török, G. (2003) *A magyar politikai rendszer*, Budapest: Osiris Kiadó.

Lijphart, A. (ed.) (1992) *Parliamentary versus Presidential Government*, Oxford: Oxford University Press.

Mihályi, P. and Molnár, L. (2006) '2006 az egészségügyi reform első szakasza', in P. Sándor, A.Tolnas and L. Vass (eds), *Magyarország politikai évkönyve 2006-ról*. I, kötet, Budapest: Demokrácia Kutatások Magyar Központja Alapítvány.

Molnár, A. (2001) 'A magyar betegjogi szabályozás a nemzetközi rendelkezések tükrében', *Lege Artis Medicinae*, 8/9: 597–610.

Pew Research (2009) 'Two decades after the wall's fall-end of communism cheered but now with more reservations', *The Pew Global Attitudes Project*, Pew Research Center, http://pewglobal.org/files/pdf/267.pdf

Sartori, G. (1976) *Parties and Party Systems. A Framework for Analysis*, Vol. 1, Cambridge: Cambridge University Press.

Sinkó, E. (2008) 'Az egészségbiztosítási rendszer átalakításának menete', in P. Sándor and L. Vass (eds), *Magyarország politikai évkönyve 2007-ről*, II, kötet, Budapest: Demokrácia Kutatások Magyar Központja Közhasznú Alapítvány.

8 Community health services in urban China: a geographical case study of access to care[1]

Yu Wang, Tanghong Jia, Jinghui Zhang, Yunli Zhang, Wen Li and Robert Haining

Introduction

Over the past sixty years, China's health care system has changed dramatically. The issue of inaccessible and expensive medical services has been increasingly debated by the domestic and international press since the mid-1990s. In order to address this pressing social issue, the Chinese government began health reforms in the early part of this century, and intensified them in 2009 by launching its most ambitious ever reform plan, including accelerating the construction of a grassroots medical system and promoting access to basic public health services. The development of a community health service system in urban areas is recognised as a key element in bringing about reform.

Given the impact that Chinese health reform could have on its people, comprising one-fifth of the world's population, as well as on its economic growth and social issues, the reform has attracted great attention and interest at home and abroad. Studies of China's health care system are not limited to medical and health policy researchers, but are also seen as important in academic fields such as sociology, anthropology and geography. This chapter aims to review the development of, and current issues in, the community health service (CHS) system that has recently been introduced in urban China, and to provide a geographical case study of access to the CHS in China's Jinan City.

The ongoing reform of China's health system

The rapid economic and industrial development taking place in China over the past three decades has been recognised globally. To a large extent, this is due to the national reform and opening-up policy that was initiated after the Cultural Revolution in the late 1970s (Chen 2002). However, since the mid-1990s the development of China's health system has largely fallen behind that of its economy, and has even been negatively influenced by economic reform that has moved the country from a planned to a market economy (Browne 2001; Eggleston et al. 2008). Despite the fact that advanced technologies are continually introduced into health services, inequality and inequity in health care have increased. Along with other important social well-being issues, such as the income and wealth gap, housing prices and government corruption, issues relating to health services are increasingly debated by the general public. According to the annual China Comprehensive Social Conditions Survey carried out by the Chinese Academy of Social Sciences, inaccessible and expensive medical services has consistently been among the top three issues of concern to the public (CASS 2011). Health care expenditure has continued to rise rapidly over the past few years – an issue regarded as important by over 42 percent of respondents.

Nevertheless, the issue of inaccessible and expensive medical services is currently misunderstood by many people. The fact is that it has become more difficult and more expensive for patients to see expert doctors in elite hospitals, in part because that is where people overwhelmingly tend to go, not that there is a general problem of lack of medical resources across the country. The problem of access to elite hospitals also reflects the poor structure of China's health system. Health care at the primary level has been much neglected, and most health services have to rely on hospitals. The problems with China's health system have emerged in tandem with the country's socio-economic development. From 1949 to the mid-1990s, the planned economy model was followed in China because of the country's limited economic strength. During this period, health care services were organised according to administrative divisions. A patient had to see a doctor in a local clinic in the first place and was not allowed to go to a district hospital directly unless the problem could not be treated at the clinic. If the problem could not be treated in a district hospital, the patient would then be referred to a hospital at the city or provincial level. Under this model, the delivery of health services was well ordered, and the usage of limited medical resources at various levels was relatively appropriate. With a market economy model replacing the planned economy in the early 1990s, the administrative boundaries of the health service system gradually disappeared, allowing freedom of choice for all patients. Understandably, people tend to prefer to see medical experts in the best hospitals, and this has contributed to the development of large hospitals in cities. More and more importance has been attached to hospital services, giving rise to a proliferation of specialists and the excessive use of drugs and high-technology diagnostic tests, whilst cost-effective primary care services have been neglected by the national health sector, health care providers and the general public. As a result, large hospitals have become overcrowded and the cost of medical services has also increased significantly. In addition, the positive consequences of economic development, such as increasing awareness of preventive health care, and of the negative consequences of industrial development, such as environmental pollution and traffic injuries, have also contributed to the population's need and demand for health services from medical experts in large hospitals. It has been widely recognised that there are two significant direct consequences of this: uneven allocation and usage of health services; and the collapse of health service providers such as small district hospitals and local clinics.

In 2003, the severe acute respiratory syndrome (SARS) epidemic played out in the glare of the international press. This was a national wake-up call that highlighted the weak state of China's public health infrastructure and the inequities in the health system. It was a turning point that led the government to begin fundamentally reforming China's health system (Shaw 2006). After a long period of internal debate and preparation, in March 2009 the Chinese government launched its most significant policy to further the reform of the health care system. This policy aims to gradually provide everyone with basic health care services and to raise the health status of the general public (State Council 2009). Five areas were identified as key for the period 2009–11: (1) accelerating the construction of the basic medical security system; (2) establishing a preliminary national essential drug system; (3) improving the grassroots medical and health care service system; (4) promoting universal access to basic public health services; and (5) advancing a pilot reform of public hospitals. The government also promised to spend an additional 850 billion renminbi (RMB) by 2011, which is about US$123 billion (Liu et al. 2011). The hope is that these efforts will bring 90 percent of China's 1.3 billion people a better health system that provides an efficient public health service, networks of improved local clinics and high quality services in public hospitals. Further, a long-term target is to establish a comprehensive primary health care system covering the entire urban and rural population by 2020. The construction of a community-based system is regarded as the cornerstone of the entire health reform plan.

Community health services in China

Primary care and community health care

Primary health care is considered by the World Health Organization (WHO) to be of crucial importance to the health of everyone. It has been suggested that up to 70 percent of people's health problems can be solved at primary care level, as opposed to secondary and tertiary care treatments and operations in hospitals (Sun 2001). Since it offers care to the largest proportion of the population, and is an important means of preventing illness as well as treating disease, the primary care sector is recognised as the most essential part of any health care system. In wealthy countries such as England, primary health care providers facilitate the provision of first-contact, comprehensive and coordinated medical care that plays a gatekeeper role in relation to hospital-based secondary and tertiary care.

The term 'community' is widely used in the literature regarding health care, especially as it concerns primary health care. Labonte (1988) defines community as 'individuals with shared affinity, and perhaps a shared geography, who organise around an issue, with collective discussion, decision-making and action'. In the context of community health care, 'a shared geography', which can be understood as the 'neighbourhood', would be a key feature of community. Although the structures and management strategies of community health care systems vary from country to country, community health care systems around the world all share a common characteristic: community health institutions provide primary health care services to people living in a defined catchment area. Primary health care in urban China is defined as the delivery of comprehensive, continuous and convenient, episodic and preventive health care services to families in the community (Bhattacharyya et al. 2011). China's primary health care model is based on the massive development of community health care in cities.

China's CHS from the 1980s to 2006

Unlike most Western European countries, where community health service systems mostly began in the early 1940s, the urban CHS system in China has a relatively short history. Fundamentally, China's CHS system is a product of a series of national policy reforms throughout the past three decades, which can be divided into three stages: the initial stage from the 1980s to 1996; the exploratory stage from 1997 to 2005; and the implementation stage from 2006 to the present (Jin et al. 2008; Hu et al. 2010).

The concept of community health care was initially introduced from the West to China in the early 1980s by a group of experts in social medicine. The initial specification was based on the functions and benefits of community health care, drawing on experiences from Western countries, the guidance for primary health care set out by the WHO, and the particular needs and conditions for developing community health care services in China. Initially, this resulted in the creation of academic primary care departments in a number of universities and medical colleges in large cities, leading to concepts of primary care and community health being gradually accepted as disciplines within the field of Chinese medical education. However, no great importance was attached to them by the government or the general public. This phase lasted for more than ten years.

The idea of developing community health services in China was first put forward by the government in late 1996, in its reform policy entitled 'Suggestions for health reform and development' (see State Council 2006). This was the first time that the term 'community health services' had ever been used in a government document at the national level. Implementing a CHS system was a brand new challenge for the central government, as it was unrealistic for China to try to imitate a community health care model from a developed country. From 1996 to 2005, China spent ten years working out a CHS model that would fit into the existing health system. A three-year nationwide trial was first launched by the Ministry of Health in order to explore the best way of setting up and operating community health institutions, as these were expected to play a major role as primary care providers. Also, a large number of community health centres and stations were rapidly set up in urban areas across China from 1997. However, the enthusiasm for developing an urban CHS lasted for only four years in many provinces, mainly due to a lack of financial support from the provincial governments and the difficulty of linking community health care with existing hospital services. But in 2003, the SARS epidemic highlighted the weak infrastructure of the national public health system and resulted in the government deciding to strengthen the development of CHS. By 2005, a rudimentary CHS system had been established across all large and medium-sized Chinese cities, as a result of which community health centres and stations were set up. But they were unable to take on the role of providing comprehensive grassroots level health care because of a series of issues including poor operating mechanisms, the limited range and quality of care, and problems with staff training.

In 2006, *Guiding Suggestions of the State Council on Developing Urban Community Health Services* was promulgated by the State Council as a top-level policy document. This was regarded as a milestone in the development of CHS in China. In contrast to the first guidance on exploring and developing CHS, released in 1997, the policy developed by the State Department in 2006 contained a range of specific strategies and targets for each province. This aimed to establish a standard CHS system. Within this policy there were a number of significant points that indicated clear directions and key areas for the development of CHS in China over the next decade. More importantly, the government's responsibility, at both national and provincial levels, for developing CHS was re-emphasised and the government started to provide financial support to local community health institutions. These policies are currently being applied across the nation.

Vision from 2006: functions and features of CHS in China

According to the reform policy released by the State Department, developing CHS is regarded as foundational to achieving primary health care covering all urban populations. The national document put forward by the State Council in 2006 clearly delineated a standard model for developing CHS in China. The functions of urban CHS were described by the governmental health sector in terms of 'six aspects in one', which refer to the six main functions of China's CHS, namely: (1) health education, (2) prevention, (3) health care, (4) rehabilitation, (5) family planning and (6) treatment services for common and frequently occurring illnesses. These are expected to be integrated to form a standard community health care system. Local households and residents constitute the recipients of CHS, with a particular focus on women, children, the elderly, patients with chronic illnesses, the disabled and the poor. The service mode of community health institutions means they will take the initiative in offering services to local residents, which is different from hospitals, and that they will gradually assume the responsibility and duties of gatekeeper with respect to residents' health care (Jin et al. 2008).

In order to establish community health institutions, local governments at provincial and city levels were required to compile development plans. The aim of these was to foster a CHS network based on community health centres and stations, complemented by other grassroots-level health institutions such as clinics and care centres. According to the State Council's policy, in principle at least one community health centre for every 30,000 to 100,000 people, or at least one within every administrative jurisdiction of various street committees (i.e. sub-district level), were to be set up in large and medium-sized cities. People living in the catchment area of a community health centre automatically become eligible for care there. Community health stations could also be established if necessary, to be managed along with community health centres. The establishment of community health institutions depends mainly on existing health resources, transformed or upgraded small hospitals and private clinics, as well as certain medical institutions affiliated to state-owned enterprises (SOEs) and public institutions (State Council 2006). By 2010, CHS had been expanded to cover over 90 percent of Chinese cities, with more than 6900 community health centres and 25,800 stations. Amongst these community health institutions, more than 60 percent were government (mainly local health sector)-run; about 30 percent were enterprise- and hospital-owned; and the remaining 7 percent were run by the private sector (MoH 2011).

It is worth pointing out two distinctive features of the CHS in China that are different from the general practice system in Western models. One is the breadth of the services the CHS now offers in the country. From health education, prevention, care, rehabilitation and family planning to treatment, the CHS in China can provide both health and some general community services via a proactive and humanistic approach, including features such as palliative care and poverty relief. This is different from the common Western model, in which general practice services mainly offer clinical health services, especially disease diagnoses and treatments, whereas a variety of public health and other types of community work are carried out by other bodies or organisations, including charities and community volunteers. The other distinctive feature is the strong presence of traditional Chinese medicine in CHS institutions, partly due to their being promoted by both central and local governments. This is mainly because of the low cost and strong preventative role of traditional Chinese medicine, which strongly correlates with the essential features of primary care at the community level. Traditional Chinese medicine differs from Western medicine mainly in its focus on individual patients rather than pathologies, and the taking into account of external natural factors such as environment, location, climate and season for diagnosis, prescription and therapy (Tang et al. 2008). At the local community level, close doctor–patient relations enhance traditional Chinese medicine in health care. In Jinan City, 32 percent of the staff in CHS institutions have either a traditional Chinese medicine education background or clinical certificates, and over 60 percent of community out-patients receive traditional Chinese medicine treatments such as herbal drug prescriptions, acupuncture, moxibustion and massage (JMHB 2011). The CHS role in community health promotion has thereby been greatly enhanced.

Current issues and challenges for China's CHS

As the Chinese CHS has been in development for only a short period, most community health institutions have not met the standard for offering comprehensive primary care services set by the State Council, especially with respect to system-initiated services and preventive health care. In contrast to the well developed National Health Service (NHS) in the UK, in which community-based clinical surgeries play a gatekeeper role for secondary and tertiary health care and act as 'first-contact care', community health care in China has not fully served as a gatekeeper in relation to secondary specialised care or other professional services. Along with the development of this, many challenges and issues relating to China's CHS system have been raised over the past few years. This section aims briefly to summarise and explore the links among these issues.

Firstly, the concept of community health care lags behind the infrastructural development of CHS institutions. For a long time, due to a less developed economy and low living standards compared with Western countries, the reactive model of health has dominated the general understanding of health care in China, focusing on diagnosis and treatment but not preventive health care. In many cities, a large proportion of people do not know of the existence of community health institutions in their own communities, and know even less about the scope of their services (Bhattacharyya et al. 2011). A majority of CHS users, including those who frequently use CHS, often see community health centres/stations as community hospitals. This reflects the fact that, although many people may make good use of the services provided by community health institutions, they do not fully understand the difference between hospitals and CHS in terms of their roles in providing primary health care. They might be excused for this, however, because many community health institutions used to be small hospitals and, indeed, follow a hospital service model in which preventive health care, chronic disease management and health education have not properly materialised. The government has begun to emphasise the primary care role of community health institutions only in the past few years, and the concept of preventive health care has still not been fully appreciated by the public. Although some first-class community health institutions have been set up in large cities, their services by local residents, especially for the preventive side of health care, may not be effective.

Secondly, resources for community health care are very limited, in terms of both quality and quantity. Since the development of community health care provision is fairly recent and the establishment of community health institutions in urban areas is still in progress, there is a great demand for general practitioners. According to the lowest acceptable standard of one general practitioner per 5000 residents, as defined by WHO, 160,000 general practitioners are needed for the 0.5 billion urban population in China. However, there were only 73,000 registered general practitioners in China in

2010, less than half the number required (MoH 2011). As stated in the reform policy in 2009, the government aimed to have an additional 60,000 trained within three years, and 300,000 within ten years. This is an ambitious plan, but essential in view of the large size of China's population (Liu et al. 2011). Furthermore, the numbers of nurses and paramedics working in community health institutions are generally low. A report showed that the doctor-to-nurse ratio in Chinese community health institutions was around 1:0.94, in contrast to the globally recognised range of 1:2 to 1:4 (Huang and Zou 2007). This shortage of nurses and paramedics has a direct impact on the range of services, as well as the quality of health care services available at the community level. For instance, community nursing for the elderly, healing and home visiting services, database management and statistics cannot be implemented effectively without sufficient numbers of nurses and paramedics.

The low quality of services in the CHS system in China is another major issue. Medical staff working in these institutions are from different backgrounds, depending on the type of community health institution in which they work (hospital-affiliated, school/factory-affiliated, transformed small hospital and/or transformed private clinic), and have different levels of qualifications. Thus the clinical skills of health workers in CHS institutions are generally lower than those found in hospitals. Unlike the well established general practitioner training system of the NHS in the UK, where doctors need to undergo at least eleven years of study and training to become qualified general practitioners after leaving school, there was no national GP qualification-authentication system in China until 2008, and even now this is only a professional development course followed by an examination, rather than a comprehensive education scheme. A number of surveys have shown that lack of public confidence in the quality of care provided in community health institutions is the main reason why people bypass them, perceiving specialist care in hospitals to be of higher quality (Yang and Yang 2009; Bhattacharyya et al. 2011). In mid-2011, a national standard GP education system, referred to as the 5+3 programme, was put forward by the State Council with the aim of establishing a GP system across the nation by 2020. GP candidates will be required to pass a five-year undergraduate-level course of study on clinical medicine followed by a three-year GP training programme. A number of universities in China have recently set up academic departments of general practice, to prepare for the launch of the 5+3 programme in September 2012. But while the improvement of China's CHS is focused on the general practitioners, there is a lack of awareness of the importance of training for other members of the CHS team, including nurses, pharmacologists and community midwives.

Thirdly, the development strategy for community health care services is not always uniform or effective, and this refers particularly to the level of government funding, and the way community health institutions in many cities are managed. Before 2006, the development of CHS boiled down to political guidance – there was no financial input from central government, and the operation of most community health institutions had to rely mainly on drug sales. The government emphasised its responsibility for 'purchasing services' in 2006 by starting to make payments to local community health institutions on a per capita basis; nonetheless, due to limited economic capacity and a large population, the actual effect was still inadequate. Although an estimated additional 330 billion RMB was invested by various levels of government in implementing health reforms from 2009 to 2011, the per capita investment was only 250 RMB per year, equivalent to 1.2 percent of the average annual income for urban residents. This figure is in sharp contrast to the high cost of medical services in China, where average medical expenditure per head in hospitals in 2010 was estimated to be 166 RMB per out-patient visit and 6200 RMB per in-patient admission (MoH 2011).

In addition, the management and development of community health institutions are not very effective. Since there was no uniform, specific or consistent policy for the development of CHS in China until 2007, the models followed have differed across the country. Nationally, some areas (provinces or cities) energetically followed guidance in developing their local CHS from 1996 onwards, whereas little effort was made in other places. Over time, this has caused significant spatial inequality and inequity in CHS across urban areas in China. This can be seen especially clearly when comparing large modern cities such as Beijing and Shanghai with the less developed cities in the West. At the scale of the individual city, the lack of a strategy for the sustainable development of CHS is sometimes striking, for example in the establishment of family health records. The purpose of this was very worthwhile, as the health sector wanted to use the database to control and manage chronic diseases better, as well as to monitor and promote the population's health in the long term. Nevertheless, in some areas there was too much emphasis on slogans and bureaucracy, and not enough attention paid to ensuring satisfactory outcomes. For example, in a few pilot cities that launched the CHS in 1997, the family health record booklet has gone through more than seven revisions over fourteen years, from initially being individually designed by each community health institution, to being standardised at district health sector level, to a later standardisation at city health sector level, to the most recent standardisation at provincial health sector level. Given that, in many areas, there was no electronic version of this booklet until recent years, and given the shortage of CHS workers, the work involved in each changeover was considerable. Only basic coverage and number of family health records set up were evaluated by the health sectors when carrying out their inspections, while actual usage was not taken into account. Moreover, within most Chinese cities there are significant differences in the accessibility and availability of community health care, mainly because there has been no health policy or strategy focusing on spatial allocation and equality of access to community health care.

In summary, the current issues and challenges facing China's community health care as discussed above are closely connected, as shown in Figure 8.1.

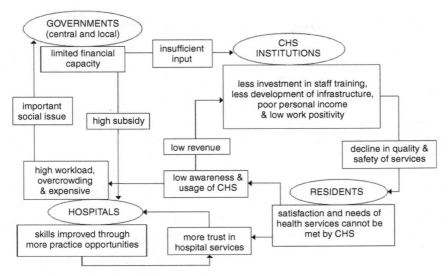

Figure 8.1 Challenges facing China's CHS system

Limited government funding and the low spending on medical training significantly restrict the ability of medical staff to treat patients, and the range and quality of services. This causes residents to distrust CHS, and so more people prefer to see doctors in hospitals than in community health institutions, even for minor illnesses (Yang and Yang 2009). In addition, doctors prefer to work in hospitals rather community health institutions – not only because hospital work generates a higher personal income, but also because as hospital doctors they gain greater respect and recognition. Since the service load of hospitals is increasing and the role of primary care in community health institutions is not widely recognised, the government allocates a higher proportion of its financial subsidy to hospitals.

The current challenges facing China's CHS are the result of a complex set of contextual factors. This includes the overall health system, which currently is not compatible with the CHS system as initially envisioned. Nevertheless, health reform, especially the reform of primary care, is an essential and intractable issue for every country in the world. Issues and challenges are unavoidable in the reform processes, but are more difficult for countries such as China that have a large population with a complex and diverse socio-economic background.

A GIS-based study of access to community health services in Jinan City

Aims of the study

Health geography provides a spatial perspective on population health, the distribution of disease in an area, and the environment's effect on health and disease. It also deals with access to health care and the spatial distribution of health care providers. Geographical information systems (GIS), which provide a set of tools for mapping and geo-analysing, have been widely used in analysing and addressing health issues, including research on primary care (Phillips et al. 2000; Yang et al. 2006). Geographers have had a long-standing interest in researching primary health care. One of the features of such health care is that it needs to be delivered locally, as many people need to use these health services relatively frequently, and it is uneconomic and in some cases impossible for would-be users to travel great distances to obtain medical advice. The catchment areas of primary care facilities tend therefore to be relatively limited in their geographical range, and the distance-decay effect on use is quite strong (Higgs 2004). Thus spatial access is particularly important for primary care services. This applies to China's CHS too, where accessibility is fundamental. Chinese community-based primary health care services seek to integrate medical care into the normal, day-to-day life space of the individual. Therefore access to CHS is a topic of great interest to health geographers and other primary health care researchers, and an important basis for evaluating the development of CHS and making suggestions for their planning and management. Since little importance has been attached to the geographical inequality of access to health care, and GIS techniques have not been widely used in health research, there have been only a very limited number of studies focusing on the accessibility and utilisation of health care services in China (Liu et al. 2007; Tao et al. 2007). This is in contrast to the large number of such studies carried out in Western countries (Luo et al. 2004; Sherman et al. 2005; Langford et al. 2008).

Geographical studies of the spatial accessibility of health care services can generally be categorised as focusing on the assessment of potential access to health services, referred to as potential accessibility; or on the analysis of the spatial utilisation of health services, referred to as revealed accessibility (Curtis 2004). Potential accessibility is often used by planners and policy analysts to evaluate an existing system of service delivery and to identify strategies for improvement. Revealed accessibility signifies the actual use of, and levels of satisfaction with, a service (Cromley and McLafferty 2002).

The present study focuses on potential accessibility to CHS in Jinan City of China. The CHS development guidelines launched by the national government in 2006 emphasised the need to provide convenient and accessible services. A target of a fifteen-minute CHS service radius for all urban populations was set by many provincial and municipal governments, including Jinan (Xian 2008). This means setting up enough community health institutions in urban areas to ensure everyone can walk to their closest CHS centre or station within fifteen minutes. Over recent years, increasing numbers of community health institutions have been set up in cities to meet this target, but limited studies have been conducted to check whether the target has been achieved. According to the Jinan Municipal Health Bureau, the CHS in Jinan has reached a coverage of 93 percent for the urban population based on local census data (JMHB

2011). In this study, we apply a GIS-based buffer-zone approach to examine this claim using the fifteen-minute service radius as the measure of potential accessibility. In addition, we identify which areas of Jinan fall within, and which areas fall outside, the fifteen-minute service area, and make a preliminary identification of the population characteristics (by housing type) of those areas lying outside.

Introduction to Jinan City

Jinan (117°00′E, 36°40′N) is the capital of Shandong Province, China, with an urban population of 2.5 million and an urban area of 1002 km². The GDP per capita in 2008 was ranked seventh out of the twenty-six provincial capital cities in China (Jinan Statistics Bureau 2009). In terms of regional administration, there are three main levels: districts, sub-districts and residential neighbourhood committee areas. Jinan City covers six districts, which contain 71 sub-districts and 424 residential neighbourhood committees within these sub-districts.

Following the first health policy, issued by the State Department in 1997, Jinan was among those cities where CHS were initially launched as a pilot. At first, community health institutions were established by affiliating them to hospitals. Between 1997 and 2006, CHS in Jinan developed rapidly as SOE-affiliated institutions and private institutions joined the system. The community health institutions in Jinan take three organisational forms, being run by either the government (61 percent), hospitals or SOEs (27 percent), or public or private institutions (11 percent). By the end of 2009, 222 community health institutions had been set up, including 62 centres and 160 stations (JMHB 2011). Community health stations in Jinan function like centres, but with a narrower range of services and fewer staff numbers.

Methodological approach

The study data consist of geographical information from the local geo-investigation centre on residential areas and locations of all the community health institutions across Jinan, as well as population census data from the local statistics bureau. An experiment was first carried out to convert the fifteen-minute walking time threshold into distance. In four selected community areas in Jinan, twenty healthy adults aged from sixteen to seventy were invited to walk from their house to the closest community health institution, based on their usual route and walking speed. The time taken for each participant was recorded and the distance travelled was measured on an E-map on a GIS platform. It was calculated that the average walking distance from house to community health institution for the twenty participants was around 800 metres. Thus, in this study, 800 metres was used as the threshold distance for a member of the general population walking towards a CHS institution for fifteen minutes. Buffer zones with an 800-metre radius from each community health institution across Jinan were created on a GIS platform. The buffer zone layer was then overlaid onto the residential areas of Jinan in order to identify those areas that were less, and those that were more than 800 metres from a community health institution. Local population census data for each residential area across the city were then used to estimate the number of people living inside and outside the 800-metre buffer zones, which reflected coverage in terms of the fifteen-minute CHS service radius. The next step was to estimate the proportion of people living inside and outside the 800-metre buffer zone in each type of residential area. The residential areas in Jinan were categorised by the Jinan Urban Planning Bureau into five types, according to the quality of housing conditions (type I – luxury low-rise houses; type II – good condition low- and high-rise buildings; type III – ordinary low- and high-rise buildings; type IV – poor condition low-rise buildings; plus a suburban/rural type). Types I–IV cover most residential areas in central urban Jinan, whereas most houses in the suburban and rural areas of the city were classified as suburban/rural. Figure 8.2 shows a map of the different types of residential area in Jinan (a) and the overlay map of the 800-metre buffer zones of community health institutions across the five types of residential area in the city (b).

Results and discussion

As shown in Table 8.1, the 800-metre buffer zones in the city cover 89 percent of the population in the central urban areas, but only 12 percent of the population in suburban/rural areas. This creates an average coverage of 74 percent in Jinan City. In other words, about 74 percent of all residents in Jinan City can reach their closest community health institution within fifteen minutes on foot, but urban residents have much better access than suburban/rural residents. Primary health care in the suburban and rural areas of Jinan City is currently being transformed from a rural basic health service system to an urban CHS system, which currently is a mixture of village clinics, township health centres and recently established community health institutions. Unfortunately, no GIS data on the locations of the village clinics and township health centres in Jinan were available for this study. Therefore, although 12 percent CHS coverage is very low, people living in suburban/rural areas may conceivably have access to primary care services through other types of service provider, such as village clinics and township clinics. Due to the lack of data and evidence, it was difficult to evaluate objectively the potential accessibility of primary care services in suburban and rural areas. Thus the focus here is on accessibility to CHS in central urban areas of Jinan.

Table 8.1 shows that service coverage in urban Jinan decreases as the quality of residential areas declines. Specifically, residential coverage in the central urban areas with type I–III housing is above 90 percent, indicating good potential accessibility to CHS.

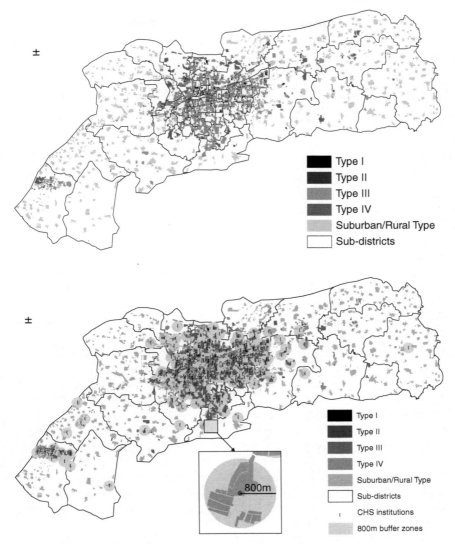

Figure 8.2 (a) Map of types of residential area in Jinan City; (b) overlay map of 800-metre buffer zones of CHS institutions in Jinan City

However, the rate decreases sharply to 76 percent in the case of poor condition low-rise buildings (type IV). The housing categories that were used in the study relate strongly to the financial situation of the residential groups in each category, and can be regarded as a proxy for socio-economic class. Hence the buffer-zone approach suggests that CHS services are more accessible for wealthier than for poorer groups. This contrasts with the fact that the need for primary health care is generally greater among poorer groups

Table 8.1 CHS 800-metre buffer zone coverage by type of residential area

	Urban area				Overall urban areas	Suburban/ rural areas	Overall Jinan City
	Type I	Type II	Type III	Type IV			
Features	Luxury low-rise houses	Good condition low- and high-rise buildings	Ordinary, low- and high-rise buildings	Poor condition low-rise buildings		Low-rise buildings	
Total population (thousands)	5.3	42.2	1773.7	207.6	2028.8	493.5	2522.3
Population outside buffer zone (thousands)	0.14	4.3	166.2	49.4	220.1	436.5	656.5
Coverage rate of 15 min CHS radius (%)	97	90	91	76	89	12	74

than among wealthier groups in the population. Along with chronically ill patients and the elderly, populations with lower incomes are the main recipients of CHS services. Therefore those living in deprived areas ideally should have priority in terms of good access to CHS compared with populations in rich areas, whereas in fact the opposite is true. This is an example illustrating the classic inverse care law – the availability of good medical care tends to vary inversely with the need for it in the population served (Hart 1971). To sum up, the assessment of potential accessibility to CHS based on a buffer-zone approach indicates that the spatial pattern of community health institutions across Jinan City is imperfect, with inequalities and inequities relating to CHS in terms of resource allocation, especially when comparing wealthy and deprived areas.

The buffer-zone approach taken in this study is a basic measure of potential accessibility to CHS, focusing only on travel distance to community health institutions in the city. Of course, physical accessibility does not guarantee utilisation, but also depends on population characteristics (Hare and Barcus 2007). For example, Haynes et al. (2003) showed that in the UK's general practice system, only 56 percent of the population of Eastern England was registered with the practice nearest their home. A simple questionnaire survey carried out alongside this GIS-based study in Jinan found that people living in type I and II residential areas generally have lower awareness of CHS and use them less than people in type III and IV areas, mainly because residents of type I and II areas tend to be wealthier and have health insurance where hospitals are the designated service providers. This suggests that, in order to optimise limited health resources and provide equitable health services to residents, the allocation of CHS resources should be closely related to the actual patterns of demand and usage of specific population groups. Future policies to improve local CHS development need to be better targeted by type for residential area. Awareness of CHS provision among people in wealthier areas whose needs are already met in other ways, should be raised. By contrast, more community health institutions are needed in poorer areas where there is a greater demand, and where people tend to make more use of CHS, but where physical access needs to be improved.

Conclusion

Compared with the well established general practice/family medicine systems in Western countries, most of which have a history of more than half a century, the CHS system in China has been formally developed for little more than ten years. Despite that fact, the CHS system is experiencing a series of issues and challenges; it is also important to recognise the advances made in recent years in terms of gradually taking on the role of primary care for urban populations, within the constraints of a situation where China is still a developing country with limited financial capacity for serving a large population. In order to overcome the existing issues and develop a comprehensive CHS system meeting the government's long-term target, an overall, well planned strategy for health care reform in China is essential. Efforts carried out in various areas (such as financial subsidies from the government, human resources management for health care, service models for community health institutions, as well as awareness of the importance of primary care) should be undertaken jointly across the whole of society. In order to put forward policy recommendations for the improvement of CHS development, a comprehensive approach from various disciplines is needed. The GIS-based study on access to CHS in Jinan City demonstrates the power of geography in evaluating access to health services. This research raises important issues regarding the optimisation of CHS resources and the equity of services, which the health sector needs to address.

Note

1 This paper is an outcome of collaborative research involving the Department of Geography at the University of Cambridge, UK and the Jinan Municipal Health Bureau in China. The project is supported by the 2010 Jinan Science and Technology Development Programme (Project No. 201003142), Jesus College, Cambridge and the Cambridge Overseas Trust. The authors thank Peggy Watson, Changming Li, K.K. Cheng, Yuyan Kong and Martin Wilkinson for helpful comments.

References

Bhattacharyya, O., Yin, D., Wong, S. and Chen, B. (2011) 'Evolution of primary care in China 1997–2009', *Health Policy*, 100: 174–80.

Browne, D. (2001) 'The long march to primary health care in China: from collectivism to market economics', *Public Health*, 115: 2–3.

CASS (2011) *The Analysis and Prediction of the Social Position in China: 2011*, Beijing: Chinese Academy of Social Science Press [in Chinese].

Chen, S. (2002) 'Economic reform and social change in China: past, present, and future of the economic state', *International Journal of Politics, Culture and Society*, 15 (4): 569–89.

Cromley, E. and McLafferty, S. (2002) *GIS and Public Health*, New York: Guilford.

Curtis, S. (2004) *Health and Inequality: Geographical Perspectives*, Los Angeles: Sage.

Eggleston, K., Li, L., Meng, Q., Lindelow, M. and Wagstaff, M. (2008) 'Health service delivery in China: a literature review', *Health Economics*, 17: 149–65.

Hare, T. and Barcus, H. (2007) 'Geographical accessibility and Kentucky's heart-related hospital services', *Applied Geography*, 27: 181–205.

Hart, T. (1971) 'The inverse care law', *The Lancet*, 297: 405–12.

Haynes, R., Lovett, A. and Sunnenberg, G. (2003) 'Potential accessibility, travel time, and consumer choice: geographical variations in general medical practice registration in Eastern England', *Environment and Planning A*, 35: 1733–50.

Higgs, G. (2004) 'A literature review of the use of GIS-based measures of access to health care services', *Health Services & Outcomes Research Methodology*, 5: 119–39.

Hu, H., Liang, W., Liu, M., Li, L., Li, Z., Li, T., Wang, J., Shi, T., Han, S., Su, M., Peng, X., Peng, Y., Zhao, W., Wang, B., Zhang, P. and Zhu, W. (2010) 'Establishment and evaluation of a model of community health service in an underdeveloped area of China', *Public Health*, 124: 206–17.

Huang, Z. and Zou, Y. (2007) 'The present situation and the countermeasures for sustainable development of community health service in China', *Chinese Journal of Social Medicine*, 24: 120–22 [in Chinese].

Jin, S., Lu, Z. and Yao, L. (2008) *Community Health Service in China*, Beijing: People's Medical Publishing House.

Jinan Statistics Bureau (2009) *Jinan Statistics Yearbook: 2008*, Beijing: China Statistic Press [in Chinese].

JMHB (2011) 'State Council's Key Contact Cities on Community Health Services – Jinan', Annual Report, Jinan Municipal Health Bureau.

Labonte, R. (1988) 'Health promotion: from concepts to strategies', *Healthcare Management Forum*, 1(3): 24–30.

Langford, M., Higgs, G., Radcliffe, J. and White, S. (2008) 'Urban population distribution models and service accessibility estimation', *Computers, Environment and Urban Systems*, 32: 66–80.

Liu, Q., Wang, B., Kong, Y. and Cheng, K. (2011) 'China's primary health-care reform', *The Lancet*, 377(9783): 2064–66.

Luo, W., Wang, F. and Douglass, C. (2004) 'Temporal changes of access to primary health care in Illinois (1990–2000) and policy implications', *Journal of Medical Systems*, 28(3): 287–99.

Liu, Z., Guo, S., Jin, H., Xie, Z., Wu, X. and Zhu, X. (2007) 'GIS-based two-step floating catchment area method in the application of spatial healthcare access in Beijing', *Science of Surveying and Mapping*, 32: 61–63.

MoH (2011) *Statistical Bulletin on the Development of Health Services in China: 2010*, People's Republic of China, Ministry of Health. www.21wecan.com/wsrcgzhyzt/wsbxw/30fd5af4bdb66d7f56ace9a732da0877.html [in Chinese].

Phillips, R., Kinman, E., Schnitzer, P., Lindbloom, E. and Ewigman, B. (2000) 'Using geographical information systems to understand health care access', *Archives of Family Medicine*, 9: 971–78.

Shaw, K. (2006) 'The 2003 SARS outbreak and its impact on infection control practices', *Public Health*, 120: 8–14.

Sherman, J., Spencer, J., Preisser, J., Gesler, W. and Arcury, T. (2005) 'A suite of methods for representing activity space in a healthcare accessibility study', *International Journal of Health Geography*. www.ij-healthgeographics.com/content/4/1/24

State Council (2006) *Guiding Suggestions of the State Council on Developing Urban Community Health Services*, State Council, People's Republic of China. www.gov.cn/zwgk/2006–02/23/content_208882.htm [in Chinese].

——(2009) *Opinions of the CPC Central Committee and the State Council on Deepening the Health Care System Reform*. www.gov.cn/jrzg/2009–04/06/content_1278721.htm [in Chinese].

Sun, Z. (2001) *Community Medicine*, Beijing: People's Health Publisher [in Chinese].

Tang, J., Liu, B. and Ma, K. (2008) 'Traditional Chinese medicine', *The Lancet*, 372: 1938–40.

Tao, H., Chen, X. and Li, X. (2007) 'Research on spatial accessibility to health service – a case study in the Haizhu District of Guangzhou', *Geomatics & Spatial Information Technology*, 30: 1–5 [in Chinese].

Xian, C. (2008) 'Constructing 15 minute service radius in Jinan', *Jinan Daily*. http://news.e23.cn/content/2008-02-12/200821200022.html [in Chinese].

Yang, D., Goerge, R. and Mullner, R. (2006) 'Comparing GIS-based methods of measuring spatial accessibility to health services', *Journal of Medical Systems*, 30(1): 23–32.

Yang, Y. and Yang, D. (2009) 'Community health service centers in China, not always trusted by the populations they serve?', *China Economic Review*, 20: 620–24.

9 'Health care and change': popular protest and building alternative visions of health systems at the end of empire

Howard Waitzkin and Rebeca Jasso-Aguilar

Although it is a complex and multifaceted phenomenon, we define empire in simple terms as the expansion beyond national boundaries of economic activities, especially investment, sales, extraction of raw materials, and the use of labor to produce commodities and services – as well as the social, political, and economic effects of this expansion. Empire has achieved many advantages for economically dominant nations. Ventures to expand empire have involved both capitalist countries and socialist superpowers (including the 'social imperialism' of the former Soviet Union). For centuries, empire included military conquest and the maintenance of colonies under direct political control. The decline of colonialism in the twentieth century, however, led to the emergence of political and economic 'neocolonialism,' by which poor countries provided similar advantages to richer countries as they had provided under the earlier, more formal versions of colonialism.

Why use the term 'empire,' rather than 'globalization'? The latter term proliferated rapidly since the early 1980s, roughly corresponding to the growth of neoliberalism as a set of policies that dominated international relations. The theory of neoliberalism argued that market exchange maximized the social good and that human well-being could advance best by enhancing individual entrepreneurial activities within the framework of strong property rights, a free market, and free trade (Harvey 2005). Neoliberalism claimed that economic growth was beneficial for everyone, at least in the long term. One of the theory's main assumptions was that economic development, accompanied by regular growth of the economy, comprised a necessary and sufficient condition to solve the problem of poverty.[1]

Beyond such economic considerations, neoliberalism also became a social, political, and cultural project (Romo 1997). Neoliberalism saw the role of the state as protecting market practices but opposed the state's roles in central planning and in the provision of public services, including medicine and public health. This opposition stemmed partly from a belief that central planning and the provision of public-sector services threatened the ability of business people and also ordinary citizens to achieve their purposes and to address social problems by exercising their personal freedom. In addition to a focus on the freedom of individuals, neoliberalism favored the free market principles of neoclassical economics, as elaborated during the second half of the nineteenth century by such figures as Alfred Marshall, William Stanley Jevons, and Leon Walras. These free market principles displaced those of the classical economic liberals, who favored a relatively but not completely unregulated market, such as Adam Smith and David Ricardo; hence the term 'neoliberal'.[2]

One crucial difference between liberalism and neoliberalism involved the latter's preference for the socialization of risk, including the risk incurred by private corporations selling health products, services, and insurance. The socialization of risk facilitated investment in uncertain enterprises by protecting investments for the investors (Harvey 2005). For instance, as in the economic crisis of the United States beginning in late 2008, the neoliberal state intervened to bail out private banks when their investments crashed. Several other terms also referred to neoliberalism: neoclassical, neoliberal, or libertarian economics; market capitalism; and market liberalism (Korten 2001). In addition, neoliberalism equated with the Washington Consensus, Reaganism, the new right agenda, corporate-led growth, and global restructuring (Korten 2001; Robinson 2004).[3]

With the growing influence of neoliberalism, globalization began to replace the terms empire and imperialism in describing the international expansion of capital. Globalization has served as an apparently more neutral term, which does not convey the exploitative and hurtful connotations of empire and imperialism. Those preferring to use the term globalization often have argued that it can refer to progressive elements of international communication, such as educational and networking activities through informational technologies, mainly the internet. Although we agree that globalized communication can achieve some fruitful consequences, we argue that the general use of the term globalization mystifies the adverse impacts that the terms empire and imperialism convey much more accurately. By focusing on the above definition of empire, which emphasizes the expansion of economic activities beyond national borders, and the social, political, and economic effects of this expansion, we call attention to the exploitative and hurtful impacts that the term globalization tends to erase. In this way, we hope to demystify, at least to some extent, the benign symbolism of globalization.

Public health and health services have played important roles in several phases of empire. The following paragraphs briefly summarize these roles. Subsequent parts of the paper analyze the decline of empire during the twenty-first century, as well as the changing roles of medicine and public health in this emerging history.

Health and the rise of empire

One basic feature of historical and contemporary empire involves the extraction of raw materials and human capital, which have moved from less developed nations to economically dominant countries. 'Underdevelopment of health' in the less developed countries follows inevitably from this depletion of natural and human resources.[4] The extraction of wealth limits poorer countries' ability to construct effective health systems. Many less developed countries also face a net loss of health workers who migrate to economically dominant nations after expensive training at home.

Through empire, corporations also have sought a cheap labor force. Workers' efficiency became one important goal of public health programs sponsored abroad by philanthropists closely tied to expanding industries in the United States. For instance, the Rockefeller Foundation's activities in public health in many countries have sought improved health conditions, especially control of infectious diseases, as a way to enhance the productivity of labor (Brown 1979). Moreover, population-control programs initiated by the United States and other dominant countries have sought more reliable participation by women in the labor force. From this rationale, a healthier, more predictable, and more productive labor force would contribute beneficially to the operations of corporations seeking to expand in less developed countries.

Another thrust of empire has involved the creation of new markets for products, including medical products, manufactured in dominant nations and sold in less developed countries. This process, enhancing the accumulation of capital by multinational corporations, has appeared nowhere more clearly than in pharmaceutical and medical equipment industries (Waitzkin 2000: ch. 4; Silverman et al. 1992; Davis 1996). The monopolistic character of these industries, as well as the stultifying impact that imported technology has exerted on local research and development, has led to advocacy for nationalized drug and equipment formularies in less developed countries, with varying success. Such advocacy also has provided a framework for resistance to trade rules that protect patents and therefore enhance the financial interests of pharmaceutical and equipment corporations operating in such countries.

Empire has reinforced international class relations, and medicine has contributed to this phenomenon. As in the United States, medical professionals in less developed countries most often come from higher-income families; even when they do not, they frequently view medicine as a route of upward mobility. As a result, medical professionals tend to ally themselves with the capitalist class – the 'national bourgeoisie' – of less developed countries. They also frequently support cooperative links between the local capitalist class and business interests in economically dominant countries (Robinson 2004, 2008). The class position of health professionals has led them to resist social change that would threaten the current class structure, either nationally or internationally (Waitzkin 2000: ch. 2).

Even after the decline of formal colonialism, empire building frequently has gone beyond economic domination to encompass some forms of military conquest. Despite its benign profile, medicine has contributed to the military efforts of European countries and the United States. For instance, health workers have assumed armed or paramilitary roles in Indochina,

Northern Africa, Iraq, and Afghanistan. Health institutions also have taken part as bases for counterinsurgency and intelligence operations in Latin America and Asia (Levy and Sidel 2008).

The connections among empire, public health, and health services have operated through several institutions that have mediated key components of these connections. Such institutions include philanthropic foundations, international financial institutions, organizations that enforce trade agreements, and international health organizations. Now we turn to each of these mediating institutions and focus mainly on their early histories. Later, we consider their more recent operations that have impacted public health and health services.

Philanthropic foundations

Although notions about beneficent contributions to the needy by wealthy people date back in western civilization to the Greek practice of 'philanthropy', modern practices that include the formation of foundations with their own legal status began in the early twentieth century, largely through the efforts of Andrew Carnegie. Having amassed a fortune in the steel industry, and already having initiated philanthropic ventures such as the Carnegie Libraries in towns throughout the United States, Carnegie developed his opinions about the social responsibilities of wealth in writings such as *The Gospel of Wealth* (Carnegie 1901).

Carnegie's book developed the principle that contributing to the needs of society was consistent with good business practice, partly to achieve favorable popular opinion about capitalist enterprises and individual entrepreneurs. By contributing intelligently to addressing social needs, rather than squandering one's wealth, Carnegie argued, the business person also could assure personal entry into the heavenly realm (thus, the framework of 'gospel'). Among the book's other notable features, Carnegie distinguished between 'imperialism' and the more virtuous 'Americanism': 'Imperialism implies naval and military force behind. Moral force, education, civilization are not the backbone of Imperialism. These are the moral forces which make for the higher civilization, for Americanism' (Carnegie 1901: 176). By creating the Carnegie Endowment for International Peace and other interconnected foundations, Carnegie acted to ensure that his beliefs achieved the fruits he preferred in the disposal of his earthly wealth and in his own heavenly future.

The most cogent early extension of philanthropic foundations to public health and health services involved John D. Rockefeller and the Rockefeller Foundation. With his fortune based in oil, Rockefeller emulated Carnegie's philanthropic activities, despite their conflicts in the realm of monopolistic business practices. However, Rockefeller and his associates moved more specifically to support public health activities and health services that would benefit the economic interests of Rockefeller-controlled corporations throughout the world.

In particular, the Rockefeller Foundation initiated international campaigns against infectious diseases such as hookworm, malaria, and yellow fever. Between 1913, the year of its founding, and 1920 the Foundation supported the development of research institutes and disease eradication programs on every continent except Antarctica. Infectious diseases proved inconvenient for expanding capitalist enterprises for several reasons, which became clear from the writings of Rockefeller and the managers of the Rockefeller Foundation (Cueto 1994; Birn et al. 2009: ch. 2). First, these infections reduced the productivity of labor by diminishing the effort that workers could devote to the job (thus the designation of hookworm, for instance, as the 'lazy man's disease'). Secondly, endemic infections in areas of the world designated for such efforts as mining, oil extraction, agriculture, and the opening of new markets for the sale of commodities made those areas unattractive for investors and for managerial personnel. Third, to the extent that corporations assumed responsibility for the care of workers, especially when workers were in short supply within remote geographical areas, the costs of care escalated when infectious diseases could not be prevented or easily treated.

To address these three problems – labor productivity, safety for investors and managers, and the costs of care – the Rockefeller Foundation's massive campaigns throughout the world fostered research and efficient delivery of services. These programs took on certain characteristics that persist to this day in some of Rockefeller's activities and also in those of other foundations, international health organizations, and non-governmental organizations. Rather than organizing 'horizontal' programs to provide a full spectrum of preventive and curative health services, the Foundation emphasized 'vertical' programs initiated by the donor that focused on a small number of specific disease entities such as hookworm or malaria. In addition, rather than broad public health initiatives to improve the economic and health conditions of disadvantaged populations, the Foundation favored the development of vaccines and medications that could prevent and treat the infectious diseases designated as most problematic – an approach some referred to as the 'magic bullet'. As shown elsewhere, these orientations have persisted in even the most recent, large-scale efforts by foundations to address public health problems in less developed countries (Waitzkin 2003; Birn 2006).

International financial institutions and trade agreements

Although trade across nations and continents dates back centuries, the framework for modern international financial institutions and trade agreements began after the Second World War with the Bretton Woods accords. These accords, which gradually emerged as an important mechanism to protect the political–economic empires of the United States and western European countries, grew from meetings in Bretton Woods, New Hampshire, that involved representatives of countries victorious in World War II.

The agreements initially focused on the economic reconstruction of Europe. Between 1944 and 1947, the Bretton Woods negotiations led to the creation of the International Monetary Fund (IMF) and the World Bank, as well as the establishment of the General Agreement on Tariffs and Trade (GATT) (Shaffer et al. 2005).

By the 1960s, after the recovery of Europe, these institutions and agreements gradually expanded their focus to the less developed countries. The World Bank, for instance, adopted as its vision statement, 'Our dream – a world without poverty'. However, because the IMF and World Bank provided most of their assistance through loans rather than grants, the debt burden of the poorer countries increased rapidly. By 1980, many less developed countries, including the poorest in the world, were spending on the average about half their economic productivity, as measured by gross domestic product, on payment of their debts to international financial institutions, even though these institutions' goals usually emphasized the reduction of poverty. These international financial institutions during the early 1980s embraced a set of economic policies known as the Washington consensus. Advocated primarily by the United States and the United Kingdom, these policies involved deregulation and privatization of public services, which added to the debt crisis by constraining even further the public health efforts and health services that less developed countries could provide.

GATT initially aimed to reduce tariffs and quotas for trade among its twenty-three member nations. The fairly simple principles of GATT included 'most favored nation treatment' (according to which the same trade rules were applied to all participating nations) and 'national treatment' (which required no discrimination in taxes and regulations between domestic and foreign goods) (Kickbusch 2000; Shaffer et al. 2005). GATT also established ongoing rounds of negotiations concerning trade agreements.

From their modest origins in GATT, international trade agreements eventually morphed into a massive structure of trade rules that would exert profound effects on public health and health services worldwide. Although we consider recent trade agreements elsewhere (Shaffer et al. 2005; Waitzkin et al. 2005), the contours of the transition from GATT to what followed proved quite dramatic. As the pace of international economic transactions intensified, facilitated by technological advances in communications and transportation, the World Trade Organization (WTO) in 1994 replaced the loose collection of agreements subsumed under GATT. The WTO and regional trade agreements have sought to remove both tariff and non-tariff barriers to trade.

Growing from the narrow scope of GATT, whose focus involved tariff barriers alone, the burgeoning array of international trade agreements encompassed under WTO expanded the purview of trade rules far beyond tariff barriers. Instead, the new trade agreements interpreted a variety of public health measures – such as environmental protection, occupational safety and health regulations, quality assurance for foods and drugs, intellectual property pertaining to patented medications and equipment, and even health services themselves – as potential barriers to trade. This perspective in trade agreements has transformed the sovereignty of governments to regulate public health and to provide health services.

International health organizations

The first approach to international public health organization evolved in Europe during the Middle Ages. At that time, some governments established local, national, and international *cordons sanitaires* – guarded boundaries that blocked people from leaving or entering geographical areas affected by epidemics of infectious diseases. In addition, governments imposed maritime quarantines that prevented ships from entering ports after visiting regions where epidemics were occurring. 'Sanitary' authorities arose mostly on an ad hoc basis and remained active mainly when epidemics were present or anticipated (Cueto 2007).

During the late nineteenth and early twentieth centuries, the rise of export economies and the expansion of economic interests worldwide triggered the demise of conventional maritime public health. Instead, the motivation for international cooperation in public health emerged largely from concerns about infectious diseases as detrimental to trade among nations that were participating in the expanding reach of capitalist enterprise. The need to protect ports, investments, and land holdings such as plantations from infectious diseases provided incentives for redesigning international public health.

The first formal international health organization arose in the Americas. Founded in Washington, DC during 1902, explicitly as a mechanism to protect trade and investments from the burden of disease, the International Sanitary Bureau focused on the prevention and control of epidemics (Cueto 2007). Mosquito eradication campaigns and the implementation of a vaccine against yellow fever occupied public health professionals in this organization throughout the early twentieth century. During that period, plans proceeded for the construction of the Panama Canal, the development of agricultural enterprises in the 'banana republics' of Central and northern South America, and the extraction of mineral resources as raw materials for industrial production from such areas as southern Mexico, Venezuela, Colombia, and Brazil. Work in the tropics demanded public health initiatives against mosquito-borne diseases such as yellow fever and malaria, parasitic illnesses such as hookworm, and the more common viral and bacterial illnesses including endemic diarrhea.

As the first modern international health organization, the International Sanitary Bureau devoted much of its early activities to infectious disease surveillance, prevention, and treatment, largely to protect trade and economic activities throughout the Americas. Later, during the 1950s, the International Sanitary Bureau became the Regional Office for the Americas of the World

Health Organization (WHO), and in 1958 changed its name to the Pan American Health Organization (PAHO). Subsequently, PAHO's public health mission broadened (Fee and Brown 2002; Cueto 2007). However, PAHO has retained a focus on the protection of trade until the present day, and in general it supports the provisions of international trade agreements.

WHO emerged in 1948 as one of the component sub-organizations of the United Nations (UN). Although prevention and control of infectious disease epidemics remained a key objective throughout its history, WHO did not frame its purpose in controlling infectious diseases as a way to protect trade and international economic transactions – as PAHO had done during its early history. Instead, during the 1970s, WHO prioritized the improved distribution of health services, especially primary health care. This orientation culminated in the famous WHO declaration on primary health care, issued at an international conference at Alma-Ata, USSR, in 1978, which provided guidelines for subsequent actions by WHO and its affiliated organizations (World Health Organization 1978; Cueto 2004; Haines et al. 2007). As the principle of universal entitlement to primary care services throughout the world became one of WHO's priorities, the organization took a strong position of advocacy on behalf of programs to improve access to care, especially in the poorest countries.

During the late 1970s and early 1980s, however, WHO entered a chronic financial crisis, produced largely because of the fragile financing provided for WHO's parent organization, the UN. Because of ideological opposition to several programs operated by component organizations of the UN, especially those of the United Nations Educational, Scientific, and Cultural Organization (UNESCO), the Reagan administration withheld from the UN large portions of the United States' annual dues. As a result, the UN began to experience increasing budgetary shortfalls, which it needed to pass on to its component organizations, including WHO. Into this financial vacuum moved the World Bank, which began to contribute a large part of WHO's budget. (The precise proportion of WHO's budget dependent on the World Bank's financing remained shielded from public scrutiny.) As its financial base shifted more toward the World Bank and away from the UN, WHO's policies also transformed to an orientation that more closely resembled those of international financial institutions and trade agreements. The financial crisis that originated in the non-payment of dues by the United States eventually led within WHO to a policy perspective regarding international trade that proved similar to PAHO's earlier orientation.

In these ways, the history of international health organizations manifested an ongoing collaboration with institutions that sought to protect commerce and trade. Constituted in the interest of trade, the organizational predecessor of PAHO devoted half a century of public health initiatives largely to the prevention and control of infections that threatened the viability of trade and investment. PAHO, and eventually WHO, sought improved health conditions in poor countries largely as a means to strengthen the economic positions of rich countries by facilitating activities that extracted raw materials and that opened new markets. The efforts of international health organizations on behalf of empire came to comprise a major focus of the public health enterprise that these organizations fostered.

Resisting empire, building an alternative future in medicine and public health

Against this historical background, conditions during the twenty-first century have changed to such an extent that a vision of a world without empire has become part of an imaginable future. Throughout the world, diverse struggles against neoliberalism and privatization illustrate the challenges of popular mobilization. In addition to these struggles *against*, groups in several countries have moved to create alternative models of public health and health services. Because empire, at least as we have known it, has ended, these efforts – especially in Latin America – have moved beyond the historical patterns fostered by capitalism and empire.

More than in Eastern Europe or in Asia, the protagonists of struggles in Latin America have experienced the direct impacts of political and economic empire imposed by the United States over the course of nearly two centuries. The policies that fortified US dominance throughout the Americas originated formally with the enunciation of the Monroe Doctrine in 1823. Subsequently, US economic and political elites succeeded in imposing a neocolonial environment, in which multinational corporations based in the United States could extract raw materials and open up new markets for the entire Western Hemisphere. The military forces of the United States protected the expanding US empire through a series of invasions and other interventions throughout the nineteenth and twentieth centuries.

Due to this long history of confronting empire, Latin America became an especially fertile ground for resistance to empire. The exploitative characteristics of empire became particularly 'knowable' in Latin America. In parallel, struggles to resist empire and to construct humane alternatives became more 'sayable' than in regions of the world with histories of exploitation somewhat less dramatic (Armony et al. 2004).

In the paragraphs that follow, we analyze a series of popular struggles in which we have been involved during the past decade as researchers and activists. These struggles include resistance against the privatization of health services in El Salvador, and efforts to expand public-sector health services in Mexico and Venezuela. Such scenarios convey a picture very different from that of the historical relation between empire and health – a picture that shows a diminishing tolerance among the world's peoples for the public health policies of empire, and a growing demand for public health systems grounded in solidarity rather than profitability.

The struggle against privatization of health services in El Salvador

One of the first outbreaks of sustained resistance to imperial policies in public health and medicine took place during the late 1990s in El Salvador. This struggle focused on privatization policies initiated by the World Bank, in collaboration with a right-wing political party that ruled El Salvador at that time. Efforts to resist privatization of health services and the public health system in El Salvador emerged as a model for analogous social movements elsewhere in Latin America. The example of El Salvador also illustrated similar processes that were to occur in many other countries throughout the world during the early twenty-first century, as imperial policies met with sustained resistance.[5]

In 1998–99, the health care sector in El Salvador fell into political turmoil when conflict broke out over various issues. First, unionized workers from the Salvadoran Institute of Social Security (*Instituto Salvadoreño del Seguro Social*, ISSS) mobilized for a salary increase in 1998, when an agreement was reached but not honored by the ISSS authorities. Second, an unfavorable revision of the collective bargaining contract in 1999 further strained the relationship between workers and the ISSS administration. And third, in 1999 the administration began to contract private entities to deliver services to the ISSS hospitals, the first signals of privatization within the ISSS. In line with this possibility, two major public hospitals under renovation remained closed for several months, waiting to have their services contracted out to private entities instead of being returned to the ISSS (STISSS 2002; Schuld 2003a).

These actions comprised part of a strategy, favored by the World Bank, to privatize public hospitals and clinics. Simultaneously, the government had tried to gather public sympathy for the privatization of health care, while avoiding the term 'privatization', on the basis of alleged corruption and inefficiency in the ISSS. Several conditions, however, called into question the credibility of such allegations. For instance, those directly responsible for the functioning of the ISSS, such as hospital directors and ISSS officials, for the previous thirteen years had been appointed by the party in power (the Republican Nationalist Alliance, *Alianza Republicana Nacionalista*, ARENA). Many ARENA politicians who supported privatization held a financial stake in the privatization effort. In addition, the health budget remained underspent, creating an artificial shortage of medications and delays in services, elements that proponents of privatization used to build the case for 'modernization' and 'democratization' of the health care system (Schuld 2003a).

These issues led to partial and temporary strikes in San Salvador. Workers mobilized on the streets where specific public hospitals were located. In November 1999, unionized workers belonging to the Union of Workers of the Salvadoran Institute of Social Security (*Sindicato de Trabajadores del ISSS*, STISSS) began a national strike – an indefinite, escalating strike. In December 1999, negotiations between the ISSS administrative authorities and STISSS workers collapsed. This collapse combined with a growing concern among doctors regarding the issue of privatization, providing the ground for an alliance between the STISSS workers and the doctors of the recently created Medical Union of Workers of the Salvadoran Institute of Social Security (*Sindicato Médico de Trabajadores del ISS*, SIMETRISSS). The medical profession, with little or no history of unionization, therefore began to join the national strike. An alliance of STISSS and SIMETRISSS produced a document labeled 'Historical Agreement for the Betterment of the National Health System' ('*Acuerdo Histórico por el Mejoramiento del Sistema Nacional de Salud*'). This document contained several points, including a key demand calling for ending privatization in the national health system: *No a la Privatización del Sistema Nacional de Salud* (SIMETRISSS 2002).

A government commitment not to privatize health services ended the conflict temporarily in March 2000. But instead of honoring the commitment, the Ministry of Health and the ISSS authorities continued to contract hospital services out to private entities, leading to an ongoing conflict that lasted until 2003 (STISSS 2002). For about three years beginning in late 1999, workers from STISSS and doctors from SIMETRISSS organized strikes and rallies that gradually drew the support of many other groups. Strikes varied in length, and participants had to walk a fine line in order not to alienate the population at large. During strikes, doctors tended to acutely ill patients on the sidewalks, a strategy as much as a humanitarian action to gain the support of the general population. Another strategic action involved 'handing the hospitals to the administrators' and walking out, a symbolic gesture to demonstrate that the hospitals could not run without doctors. The government responded with repression, using tear gas, rubber bullets, and high-pressure water against strikers; doctors were fired and replaced with new personnel (STISSS 2002).

This solidarity and organization resulted, during November 2002, in Congressional approval of Decree 1024 (Decree of State Guarantee of Public Health and Social Security, *Decreto de Garantía Estatal de la Salud Pública y la Seguridad Social*). President Francisco Flores threatened to veto the decree, but legislative pressure in Congress and civil society pressure through street demonstrations forced him to comply with it. Besides guaranteeing that health care would remain public, the decree effectively voided any health care-related contract that the government had signed with the private sector since the beginning of the conflict (SIMETRISSS 2002). But this victory was shortlived because the party in power, ARENA, formed an alliance that produced enough votes during December 2002 to repeal Decree 1024. The conflict continued for months, with several more marches and demonstrations taking place in San Salvador. These were massive rallies where demonstrators dressed in white as a symbol of peace and as a sign of solidarity with doctors and nurses wearing white gowns. The demonstrations drew from 25,000 to 200,000 participants – in a city of about 800,000 people. Many doctors sold their homes, cars, and home appliances to obtain the financial means for continuing the struggle (SIMETRISSS 2002; STISSS 2002).

The nine-month-old strike ended with a decision by the World Bank to reverse a privatization clause in a loan earmarked for modernizing the public health system. On June 13, 2003, union leaders and government representatives reached an agreement to halt the privatization of the public health system. All the members of STISSS and SIMETRISSS were reinstated under previous conditions of salaries and seniority. The agreement also called for the establishment of a commission to follow up on reforms of the health care system. The commission included medical professionals, government officials, and representatives of unions and civil society (Schuld 2003b). Efforts to maintain and to expand public-sector health care have continued, especially after the election in 2009 of left-oriented Mauricio Funes as President.

Social medicine coming to power in Mexico City

Bold new health policies, linked to the election of a progressive government in the Federal District of Mexico City, illustrate what an alternative vision of the possible can accomplish under conditions of broad sociopolitical change. In the election of 2000, the left-oriented Party of the Democratic Revolution (PDR) gained control of the government in the Federal District of Mexico City, which comprises the equivalent of a state, while the conservative Party of National Action (PAN) won the presidential election. Thus political life in Mexico during the first decade of the twenty-first century saw the strengthening of two very distinctive political and economic projects: an anti-neoliberal position in Mexico City, represented by Andrés Manuel López Obrador (known popularly as 'AMLO'), and a neoliberal one at the federal level, embodied by President Vicente Fox. The two projects led to very different results.

As governor, AMLO initiated wide-ranging reforms of health and human services. To the post of secretary of health, López Obrador appointed Cristina Laurell, a widely respected leader of Latin American social medicine (Waitzkin et al. 2001a, 2001b; Laurell 2003). Laurell and colleagues began a series of ambitious health programs, modeled according to social medicine principles. They first focused on senior citizens and the uninsured population, with a goal of guaranteeing the constitutional right to health protection.

The fourth article of the Political Constitution of Mexico and the thirty-fifth article of the federal health legislation grant this right, as well as universal coverage and free care through public institutions. However, because these documents do not clarify what entity has obligation to provide health services, this right in practice often comes to be seen as merely 'good intentions'. On the other hand, an assumption underlying these documents is that public institutions should provide health protection. This assumption provides a legal justification to make the State – presumably the guardian of public interest – the provider of this right (Laurell 2007, 2008). The Mexico City Government (MCG) made use of this legal justification to design and implement health and human services policies that targeted vulnerable groups, thus making 'the right to health protection a reality' (Laurell 2008). Broad goals that guided the MCG's approach to health policy were:

> To democratize health care, reducing inequality in disease and death and removing economic, social, and cultural obstacles to access; to strengthen public institutions as the only socially just and economically sustainable option granting equal and universal access to health protection; to attain universal coverage; to broaden services for the uninsured population; to achieve equality in access to existing services; and to create solidarity through fiscal funding and the distribution of the costs of disease among the sick and the healthy.
>
> (Laurell 2003)

Health policies of the MCG derived from a concept of social rights. Leaders of the MCG saw the creation of social rights – those that the State is required to guarantee – as one of the Mexican Revolution's most important gains (Laurell 2003).

Two major programs initiated by the MCG aimed to improve public health and medical services. First, the Program of Food Support and Free Drugs for Senior Citizens created a social institution that granted all senior citizens a new social right. This program started in February 2001, and by October 2002 it had become virtually universal, covering 98 percent of Mexico City residents aged 70 years or more. Citizens receive a monthly stipend amounting to the cost of food for one person (the equivalent of US$70) and free health care at the city government's health facilities (Laurell 2003: 30).

A second initiative, the Program of Free Health Care and Drugs, focused on uninsured residents of Mexico City. By December 2002, about 350,000 among the 875,000 eligible families had enrolled. Later, by the end of 2005, 854,000 family units had registered in the program, which effectively amounted to universal coverage of the target population. The program covered all personal and public health services; MCG health facilities offered primary and hospital care for individuals and families (Laurell 2008).

Financing these programs proved possible due to the MCG's commitment to curb administrative waste and corruption. An austerity program beginning in 2000 implemented a 15 percent pay cut for top government officials and eliminated superfluous expenses. AMLO explained these changes under the widely quoted slogan, 'We can pay for these services because the government isn't robbing you anymore.' The austerity measures yielded savings of US $200 million in 2001 and $300 million in 2002. Simultaneously, the government undertook crackdowns against tax evasion and financial corruption. These savings allowed the government to increase the health budget by 67 percent, meaning that 12.5 percent of the Mexico City budget went for public health and health services (Laurell 2008).

Such community-oriented initiatives achieved wide admiration and con-tributed to the electoral successes of the Party. While in 2000 the PRD victory in Mexico City had been tight, by April 2003 the approval rate for AMLO reached an unprecedented 80–85 percent. The PRD swept the 2003 mid-term election and took control of the Mexico City legislature.

After AMLO narrowly lost the national presidential election during 2006 – an election that generated wide dispute and that showed extensive evidence of fraud – the 'Legitimate Government of Mexico' took office. In this parallel, unofficial government, AMLO served as President, and Laurell became the Minister of Health. The parallel government kept the social medicine vision alive as a viable policy alternative. According to Laurell, the Legitimate Government of Mexico 'is not a shadow government understood as a reaction to official actions of the other government … [it is] much more proactive, [with the capacity] to elaborate and discuss original proposals using as a starting point another idea of what we want our nation to be' (Laurell 2007).

On the other hand, the Popular Insurance (*Seguro Popular*), the federal health coverage program proposed and partly implemented by Vicente Fox's administration between 2003 and 2006, comprised a service package with limited coverage, cost-sharing by families, and gradual enrollment of the uninsured population. Limited coverage disrupted the provision of comprehensive care. Cost-sharing amounted to 6 percent of family income, a financial burden for poor families. Services not included had to be purchased through private insurance (Laurell 2008). The latter signaled a further push toward the privatization of health care, which was in line with Fox's neoliberal agenda.

The different ways in which Fox and AMLO treated public health and health services policies illustrated two discrepant visions of development. In 2006, the Mexican presidential election became so contested because it served as a kind of referendum on these different projects with the potential to create very different countries. As Laurell notes:

> In 2006 what was at play was not just the election of a candidate, the future of the country was at stake … we lost the opportunity to rebuild our country and to make it less unequal, of building a nation for everyone, in which social rights are guaranteed and built, that is what we lost with this electoral fraud … What we are trying to do with the Legitimate Government and with the mobilization of citizens is to keep the hope alive.
> (Laurell 2007)

Mexico City's example of enhanced public-sector services and the Legitimate Government's enduring program for change conveyed a vision of an alternative future that will continue to inspire, within Mexico and elsewhere, during the post-empire era.

Other examples of a new vision: Venezuela, Uruguay, and Brazil

Although we have focused attention on El Salvador and Mexico City, the emergence of alternative visions and policies that do not accept the historical assumptions of empire and neoliberalism has occurred worldwide. Among many examples, recent events in Venezuela, Uruguay, and Brazil provide a multifaceted picture of new approaches to public health and medicine. The cumulative experience of such efforts during the early twenty-first century convey an overall impression that the historical linkages among empire, medicine, and public health have dissolved and that this emerging trajectory will prove difficult to reverse.

Under the presidency of Hugo Chávez, Venezuela enacted path-breaking innovations based on social medicine principles. Influenced partly by social medicine leaders such as María Urbaneja, Francisco Armada, and Oscar Feo (the first two serving as national ministers of health), the country embarked on a far-reaching series of organizational changes (Muntaner et al. 2008; Briggs and Mantini-Briggs 2009).

Although Chávez and his government advocated accessible, public-sector health services as part of its program after winning the national election in 1999, several barriers stood in the way of achieving that vision. First, the Ministry of Health in the Chávez government continued to operate in a top-down, bureaucratic manner that impeded outreach to underserved urban and rural communities. Secondly, the Venezuelan medical profession opposed proposals to expand public-sector services.

In the impasse, the *Libertador* municipality within the boundaries of Caracas initiated a grassroots effort to improve services for the poor. The municipality issued a call for physicians to live and to work in the community. When only a small number of Venezuela doctors responded, the municipality's mayor, Freddy Bernal, approached the Cuban embassy. Within several months, a contingent of Cuban doctors arrived.

This approach spread throughout Venezuela. The name of the initiative, *misión barrio adentro* ('mission of the barrio within') refers to the grassroots, bottom-up emergence of a parallel public-sector health system. Low-income communities throughout the country organized to provide their own health services, with the assistance of more than 20,000 primary care physicians from Cuba. Communities constructed their own health facilities and designed services that addressed the perceived needs of specific neighborhoods. These changes have occurred with some support but for the most part independently from the national Ministry of Health. *Misión barrio adentro* later attracted attention as a model for change in many other Latin American countries, particular in Bolivia under the presidency of Evo Morales.

After the election in 2004 of Tabaré Vázquez, an oncologist, Uruguay also has initiated dramatic reforms influenced by Latin American social medicine. In particular, a decentralization of health institutions guided by extensive neighborhood participation integrated health services with local governments at the level of the municipality. These changes occurred with the leadership of Miguel Fernández, a social medicine scholar and teacher who served as sub-secretary in the Ministry of Health. During the Vázquez Presidency, public-sector services received prioritization, and the neoliberal model fell into decline, for instance, as Uruguay refused to participate in a new free trade agreement initiated by the United States. In November 2009, Uruguayan voters elected José Mujica, a former guerilla leader, as Vázquez's successor. Mujica promised to maintain Vázquez's economic policy orientation and vowed to strengthen even further Uruguay's public-sector health services.

'Collective health', the term that characterized social medicine in Brazil, profoundly affected health policies under the government of Luiz Inácio Lula da Silva, a former trade unionist elected in 2002 and again in 2006 to two successive terms as president. Leaders of collective health participated as activists within the Workers' Party and contributed to many of Lula's electoral and substantive accomplishments. Several leaders of collective health served as influential officials in the national Ministry of Health. In local municipalities, collective health activists worked in such efforts as community-determined budgets to address local needs. Due to anticipated adverse effects on health and health services, some collective health leaders opposed Lula's policies that favored the interests of international financial capital, including the renewal of agreements with the IMF. On the other hand, Lula has received wide praise for his support of policies to strengthen public-sector services and for his willingness to oppose US policies in such venues as the WTO.

Struggles for national health programs in the heart of empire

Since at least the 1920s, during the midst of empire past, people in the United States have organized in support of a national health program that would provide universal access to comprehensive medical services. In Europe, these struggles began even earlier. For instance, in 1883, Germany became the first country in the world to establish a national health program, as part of Otto von Bismarck's social legislation that largely aimed to prevent a more wide-reaching social revolution. Although many initiatives have tried to privatize the European national health programs in part or in whole, these efforts have achieved little lasting success.[6]

Managed care evolved in the United States during the 1990s with an initial cycle of tremendous expansion and then a notable contraction. The term 'managed care' refers to health care services under the administrative control of large, private organizations, with 'capitated' financing (a prepayment of a negotiated sum of money to the managed care organization (MCO) by an employer, public agency, family, or individual per covered person per unit of time, typically a month). Beyond the capitation fee, people covered under managed care almost always pay additional co-payments when they actually receive services. By the mid-1990s, most insured persons in the United States and many other countries came to be covered by managed care organizations.

As the domestic market became more contentious and less attractive, a transition from national to multinational managed care occurred. US and European multinational corporations, including pharmaceutical companies and MCOs, turned to international markets in seeking alternative sources of profit (Price et al. 1999). Corporations exported managed care as the main organizational format, as opposed to other forms of commercial insurance, because managed care had become the dominant form of health care organization in the United States and had emerged as a profitable framework for commercial organizations to provide health insurance.

As MCOs set their sights on foreign markets, Europe initially looked promising. Reforms in several European national health programs introduced principles of managed care, market competition, and the privatization of public services (Glaser 1993; Jacobs 1998). These reforms, as components of neoliberalism, received strong support from the Thatcher government in Britain, as well as varying degrees of enthusiasm from conservative parties in other countries. Alain Enthoven and his disciples, who orchestrated the managed care proposals that shaped the Clinton Administration's ill-fated efforts for a national health program in the United States, served as consultants for European governments undertaking these reforms (Enthoven and van de Ven 2007).

The popularity of public-sector programs in Europe, however, proved a powerful disincentive to privatization. After the mid-1990s, especially as managed care became increasingly unpopular in the United States, European countries such as the United Kingdom, the Netherlands, and Sweden reversed some (but not all) policies that attempted to privatize their national health programs (Light 1997; Mackintosh and Koivusalo 2005). Although debates about privatization and 'marketization' of the European national health programs continued during more recent years, such debates in general did not lead to basic changes in the systems' fundamentally public character (Hermann 2009). With increasing saturation of markets in the United States and with limited prospects in Europe, US-based MCOs turned to less developed countries, especially in Latin America. US corporations exported, in the form of managed care, products and practices that had come under heavy criticism domestically – as some pointed out, in the tradition of tobacco and pesticides (Waitzkin 2011). The export of managed care received enthusiastic support from the World Bank, other international financial institutions, and multinational corporations. On the receiving end, less developed countries experienced strong pressure to accept managed care as the organizational framework for privatization of their health and social security systems. MCOs and investment funds rapidly entered the Latin American market, and this experience served as a model for the export of managed care to Africa and Asia (Stocker et al. 1999).

In the United States, the latest of many attempts to achieve a national health program involved President Barack Obama's efforts, which resulted during March 2010 in the passage of the highly contested Patient Protection and Affordable Care Act. Earlier in his career, Obama had supported a single-payer, public-sector program of universal health care. However, in his Presidential campaign of 2008, he received approximately three times more contributions from the private for-profit insurance industry than did his Republican Party opponent, John McCain. Unsurprisingly, the Patient Protection and Affordable Care Act called for the preservation and strengthening of the private insurance industry through vastly increased public payments to the industry for the care of uninsured and underinsured people.[7]

Despite the complexity of the Patient Protection and Affordable Care Act, its basic components resembled those of many health reform proposals favored by international financial institutions and multinational insurance corporations throughout the world during empire present. Such proposals aimed to enhance access by corporations to public-sector health and social security trust funds. An ideology favoring for-profit corporations in the marketplace justified these reforms through unproven claims about the efficiency of the private sector and about enhanced quality of care under principles of competition and business management. Such reforms usually dealt with health care as a commodity to be bought and sold in a competitive marketplace, rather than as a fundamental human right to be guaranteed by government according to the principle of social solidarity.

The contrast between a single-payer approach versus the Patient Protection and Affordable Care Act resembles the contrast between public-sector versus market-based reform proposals that occurred worldwide during empire present. As noted, political and economic elites supported market-based reform as a route to enhance investment opportunities and profitability for multinational corporations selling private health insurance, medications, and equipment. Advocated by the leadership of those corporations and international financial institutions such as the World Bank, these market-based proposals sought to use public-sector funds, usually in the target countries' social security systems, to subsidize private-sector corporate expansion.

Like many national health programs around the world, a single-payer program in the United States basically would extend Medicare to the entire population. Although Medicare has not been without problems, people over sixty-five years of age have widely supported the system and have expressed satisfaction with it. Under Medicare, the government occupies a very small role. The government collects payments from workers, employers, and Medicare recipients and then distributes funds to health care providers for the services that Medicare patients receive. Because it is such a simple system, the administrative costs under Medicare average between 3 and 5 percent, according to most studies. This small percentage means that the vast majority of Medicare expenditures pay for clinical services as opposed to administrative expenses.

On the other hand, private insurance generally shows administrative expenses between 20 and 30 percent (Woolhandler et al. 2003), and there is little evidence that administrative waste will decrease substantially under the Patient Protection and Affordable Care Act. This much larger percentage means that about one quarter of every dollar spent on health care goes for administrative costs. Many of these expenditures pay for activities such as billing, denial of claims, supervision of co-payments and deductibles, scrutiny of pre-existing conditions that disqualify people from care (the Patient Protection and Affordable Care Act would prohibit such practices based on pre-existing conditions, but the prohibition would be phased in over a period of years), and exorbitant salaries for executives (in some cases totaling between \$10 and 20 million per year).

A single-payer national health program would achieve universal access to care by drastically reducing administrative waste.[8] All people would receive the care that they need without co-payments, deductibles, or other expenses at the point of service. Under a single-payer system, the average family and the average business would spend the same or less than they previously spent on medical expenses. Despite lack of support by the Obama Administration and many Congressional representatives, national polls consistently have shown that a majority or plurality (depending on the poll) of people in the United States have favored the single-payer approach.[9]

The Obama administration's proposal, as well as the highly modified Patient Protection and Affordable Care Act (which eventually passed Congress by a narrow majority as part of the budget reconciliation process rather than as stand-alone legislation), involved a 'mixed' approach to linking the public and private sectors. In the mixed model, private health insurance corporations receive public-sector funds, deriving mostly from tax revenues. These funds subsidize private insurance, which insurance corporations continue to administer. Although the Obama administration also proposed a 'public option,' to be operated by the federal government, Obama eventually dropped the public option, largely due to opposition from the private insurance industry and from the industry's supporters in Congress.[10]

As a result of this process, the overall national health program, as enacted in the Patient Protection and Affordable Care Act, retained the previous private insurance industry as the main administrative entity, and therefore projected a much higher level of administrative costs than a single-payer approach. Because the mixed approach would not significantly reduce administrative waste, the anticipated costs of the proposal predictably would become prohibitive, despite assurances to the contrary. Concern about these high costs became a key focus of debate in Congress and throughout the United States. Moreover, even in the best-case scenario, the Patient Protection and Affordable Care Act would leave nearly one-half of the previously uninsured population, about 23 million people, still uninsured.[11]

Obama and his core staff members consistently argued that it was important to preserve the for-profit private insurance industry, with even more tax subsidies for the industry. The Patient Protection and Affordable Care Act essentially would compel families and individuals to buy insurance from the private industry, with the poor assisted through a means-testing approach requiring huge administrative costs. In prior state-level programs that involved a mixed private and public approach, these programs failed to achieve universal coverage and generated crippling cost overruns (for instance in Massachusetts, frequently cited as a model for the Obama proposal) (Woolhandler et al. 2008).

Other countries that have implemented mixed private–public systems have encountered challenging problems. Although some European systems have received critical attention (Bodenheimer and Grumbach 2009; Reid 2009), several middle-income countries in Latin America also have tried to implement mixed systems. These initiatives were largely due to the requirements of international financial institutions such as the World Bank and IMF, which demanded a reduction of public-sector services and an expansion of private-sector services as a requirement of new or renegotiated loans (Waitzkin et al. 2007).

In these countries, neither the conversion of public-sector to private-sector insurance, nor the expansion of private insurance through enhanced public financing and participation by corporate entrepreneurs, succeeded in assuring access to needed health services. Expansion of private insurance often generated additional co-payments. Privatization of social security and other public-sector trust funds for health services generally favored private corporations by providing publicly subsidized insurance and by increasing the capital held by these corporations. In addition, privatization led to higher administrative costs.

The impact of mixed private–public systems varied across countries. For Argentina, these policies led to increasing economic crisis and major cutbacks of services, especially for older and disabled people. In Chile, where privatization occurred largely during the military dictatorship, private MCOs (subsidized by public tax funds) prospered as they covered relatively healthy groups in the population, while a constricted public sector continued to provide services to the uninsured. Mexico faced pressures from the World Bank to privatize its social security system, including public-sector health services; as avenues opened to the participation of private corporations, public-sector institutions encountered budget reductions that led to eroded services.

If we are serious about working to improve the devastating problems of access to services in the United States and other countries, we need to move beyond conventional wisdom about the positive impact of market-based policies such as mixed private–public systems. Strategies that channel public funds into private insurance corporations have failed to achieve the goal of universal access. Unfortunately, such policies may worsen even further the conditions faced by vulnerable groups. Based on empirical realities, our work must find ways to enhance the delivery of public-sector services, rather than continuing to implement the mostly failed policies of privatization. In the United States, the center of empire present, these failed policies will continue to exhaust the already fragile national economy, while leaving a large part of the population with inadequate access to services.

Because the Patient Protection and Affordable Care Act very likely will fail to achieve its purposes of universal access and cost control, organizing to achieve a public-sector national health program based on single-payer principles will continue.[12] As the United States remains the only economically advanced country without a viable national program that assures access to needed care, the single-payer approach will come to be seen as the only way to avoid the failures that have plagued the country for so many years. In the long run, we might take hope from Winston Churchill's much quoted observation, 'The United States invariably does the right thing, after having exhausted every other alternative.'[13]

Health care and change at the end of empire?

At the end of the twentieth century, trade agreements were strengthening the political and economic positions of the United States and other dominant nations in North America and Europe, but the twenty-first century has seen a rapid deterioration of this mechanism of empire building and maintenance. As only one key example, collective actions led to the failure of attempts to pass the Free Trade Area of the Americas, an agreement that would have converted the western hemisphere into one free trade zone, along the lines of the North American Free Trade Agreement. With rare exceptions such as the Dominican Republic–Central American Free Trade Agreement, similar actions have forced the US government to implement bilateral free trade agreements sporadically with single countries, instead of reaching regional agreements that could achieve compliance to imperial principles by a wider spectrum of countries.

The collapse of the WTO's round of negotiations in 2008 implied the probable end of US and Western European hegemony in trade agreements. This collapse resulted from resistance (partly to agricultural tariffs) by an emerging coalition: the Common Market of the South in Latin America (Mercosur, led by Brazil and also involving Argentina, Paraguay, Uruguay, and Venezuela as full members), China, and India. This transition will continue to change profoundly the prior adverse effects of trade agreements on public health and health services.

Alternative trade agreements, not involving the United States or Western European countries, have emerged.[14] The first such agreement in Latin America was the Mercosur. Another, increasingly influential agreement is the Bolivarian Alliance for the Peoples of Our America (*Alianza Bolivariana para los Pueblos de Nuestra América*, ALBA). Initiated by Venezuela, ALBA includes Cuba, Bolivia, Nicaragua, Ecuador, Dominica, Saint Vincent and the Grenadines, and Antigua and Barbuda. These alternative trade agreements create collaborative trade activities that minimize the dominant and often exploitative efforts previously exerted by the United States and other countries of the 'North'. Several of the agreements involve cooperation in public health and medical care, such as Cuba's sending physicians to work in Venezuela and Bolivia in exchange for oil and natural gas.

Considering only Latin America, progressive governments have come to power as a result of electoral victories in Venezuela, Ecuador, Bolivia, Chile,

Argentina, Uruguay, Brazil, Nicaragua, Honduras, Paraguay, El Salvador, and Peru.[15] These governments generally have rejected the historical principles and relationships associated with empire. Several of the countries (particularly Venezuela and Bolivia) have explicitly adopted visions of a peaceful, electoral transition to socialism – a transition that imperial powers previously would not have tolerated, as in the case of Chile during the early 1970s. Empire's deterioration has carried with it a reduced capacity to destroy democratically elected governments that do not defer to imperial expectations. One key policy that typically characterizes such new governments involves a reversal of neoliberal requirements for the reduction of public-sector health services and, instead, a strengthening of those services.

The weakness of capitalist empire in response to these changes became clearer after 2008, with a near collapse of the international capitalist banking system; the socialization through increased government ownership of banks and other large private enterprises such as the auto industry; and the over-extension and ineffectuality of military operations. So far, the expansion of government ownership in the capitalist economy has continued to benefit mainly the rich. But the debility revealed by actions to socialize increasing parts of the capitalist economy became inescapably clear to any who cared to look closely. Likewise, the prospect of endless war, usually perpetrated in the name of anti-terrorism, uncovered the underlying desperation of 'disaster capitalism' (Klein 2007). This stage of capitalism maintains itself largely by creating disasters through war so that corporate actors can open new markets and opportunities for investment by strengthening 'security' and reconstructing war-torn societies.

Such changes hearken back to prediction of the ever-controversial V. I. Lenin, whose stature as an analyst of capitalism's vulnerability during the era of empire has grown as more recent analysts such as Chalmers Johnson and Johan Galtung have reached similar conclusions (Lenin 1917 [1963]; Johnson 2004a, 2004b, 2006; Galtung 2009).[16]

Sociomedical activism in the post-empire era

The struggles considered here confirm certain core principles of public health: the right to health care, the right to water and other components of a safe environment, and the reduction of illness-generating conditions such as inequality and related social determinants of ill health and early death. Affordable access to health care and clean water supplies provided by the state, for instance, has become the focus of activism throughout the world. Such struggles reaffirm the principle of the right to organize at the grassroots and to have communities' voices heard and counted in policy decisions. This activism fosters a sense of dignity associated with citizenship. Activism that seeks alternatives to neoliberalism and privatization encourages participation by diverse populations, an emphasis on solidarity, and a rejection of traditional political forms. Reinforcing this view, Pierre Bourdieu places such new social movements at the heart of the struggle against neoliberalism, as the state and civil society transform (Bourdieu 2003).

As William Robinson argues, such popular struggles and organized resistance respond to the exploitative practices of global capitalism and empire, but also move beyond those practices. He situates these struggles within the context of the transnational state, noting that 'the challenge is how to reconstruct the social power of the popular classes worldwide in an era in which such power is not mediated and organized through the nation state' (Robinson 2004). From this perspective, mass mobilization by civil society opens counter-hegemonic spaces, in which the given wisdoms that foster empire become demystified and unacceptable.

The challenge is to develop strategies for activism that can extend these counter-hegemonic spaces to broader social change. A goal of the social movements that we have described is not simply to win, but also to encourage public debate and to raise the level of political consciousness. This new consciousness rejects the inevitability of empire and also fosters a vision of medicine and public health constructed around principles of justice rather than commodification and profitability. As the era of empire passes, no other path will fulfill our most fundamental aspirations for healing.

Notes

1 For further perspectives on the impact of neoliberalism in medicine and public health, see Kim et al. (2002); Fort et al. (2004); Navarro (2007); Panitch and Leys (2009). In this chapter, we refer to themes developed further in Waitzkin (2011).

2 Pertinent sources include Smith (1776 [1904]); Ricardo 1817 [1971]; Jevons (1911 [1970]); Marshall (1920 [1997]); Walras (1984).

3 For a complementary slant on these distinctions, see Hunter and Yates (2002).

4 This perspective was first argued by Navarro (1974).

5 Observations in the sections on El Salvador, Bolivia, and Mexico derive from the participatory field work of Rebeca Jasso-Aguilar and the sources cited below.

6 For a helpful comparative overview of national health programs in Europe and elsewhere, see Reid (2009).

7 A summary and major components of the US health reform legislation appear in 'Understanding the patient protection and affordable care act', www.healthcare. gov/law/introduction/index.html. For information about Obama's switch from single-payer to market-oriented principles and the campaign contributions that supported this conversion, see: 'Barack Obama on single payer in 2003', www. pnhp.org/news/2008/june/barack_obama_on_sing.php; and Jacobson (2010).

8 Physicians for a National Health Program, 'Single-payer national health insurance', www.pnhp.org/facts/single_payer_resources.php

9 Western Pennsylvania Coalition for Single-Payer Healthcare, 'Single-payer poll, survey, and initiative results', www.wpasinglepayer.org/PollResults.html; Healthcare-Now!, 'Another poll shows majority support for single-payer', www.healthcare-now. org/another-poll-shows-majority-support-for-single-payer

10 The White House, 'The Obama Plan: stability and security for all Americans', www.whitehouse.gov/issues/health-care

11 'Health Bill leaves 23 million uninsured', http://pnhp.org/news/2010/march/pro-single-payer-doctors-health-bill-leaves-23-million-uninsured

12 Physicians for a National Health Program, 'Single-payer national health insurance', www.pnhp.org/facts/single-payer-resources; Healthcare-Now!, 'Organizing for a national single-payer healthcare system', www.healthcare-now.org

13 Winston Churchill, 'Collected quotations, unsourced', http://en.wikiquote.org/wiki/Winston_Churchill

14 Membership in the alternative trade agreements was current as of July 2010.

15 These electoral victories were current as of July 2010. In Chile a conservative candidate, Sebastián Piñera, gained the presidency in March 2010 by a narrow margin, after progressive President Michelle Bachelet, whose popular support was 84 percent at the end of her term according to polls, could not run due to a constitutional two-term limit. Bachelet did not rule out a presidential candidacy in 2014. www.nasdaq.com/aspx/stock-market-news-story.aspx?storyid=201003090924dowjonesdjonline000277&title=chile-president-bachelet-maintains-84-approval-after-earthquake-poll

References

Armony, V., Lamy, P. and Tremblay, A. (2004) *Values, Culture, and the Economic Integration of Latin America and North America: An Empirical Perspective on Culturalist Approaches*, Diálogos Latinoamericanos No. 9, Aarhus, Denmark: Center for Latin American Studies, Aarhus University.

Birn, A.-E. (2005) 'Gates's grandest challenge: transcending technology as public health ideology', *The Lancet*, 366: 514–19.

Birn, A.-E. (2006) *Marriage of Convenience: Rockefeller International Health and Revolutionary Mexico*, Rochester, NY: Rochester University Press.

Birn, A.-E., Pillay, Y. and Holz, T.H. (eds) (2009) *Textbook of International Health: Global Health in a Dynamic World*, New York: Oxford University Press.

Bodenheimer, T.S. and Grumbach, K. (2009) *Understanding Health Policy: A Critical Approach*, Stamford, CT: Appleton & Lange.

Bourdieu, P. (2003) *Against the Tyranny of the Market*, London: Verso.

Briggs, C. and Mantini-Briggs, C. (2009) 'Confronting health disparities: Latin American social medicine in Venezuela', *American Journal of Public Health*, 99: 549–55.

Brown, E.R. (1979) *Rockefeller Medicine Men: Medicine and Capitalism in America*, Berkeley, CA: University of California Press.

Carnegie, A. (1901) *The Gospel of Wealth and Other Timely Essays*, New York: The Century Company.

Cueto, M. (ed.) (1994) *Missionaries of Science: The Rockefeller Foundation and Latin America*, Bloomington, IN: Indiana University Press.

——(2004) 'The origins of primary health care and selective primary health care', *American Journal of Public Health*, 94: 1884–93.

——(2007) *The Value of Health: A History of the Pan American Health Organization*, Rochester, NY: Rochester University Press.

Davis, P. (ed.) (1996) *Contested Ground: Public Purpose and Private Interest in the Regulation of Prescription Drugs*, Oxford: Oxford University Press.

Enthoven, A. and van de Ven, W.P. (2007) 'Going Dutch – managed-competition health insurance in the Netherlands', *New England Journal of Medicine*, 357: 2421–23.

Fee, E. and Brown, T.M. (2002) '100 Years of the Pan American Health Organization', *American Journal of Public Health*, 92(12): 1888–89.

Fort, M., Mercer, M.A. and Gish, O. (eds) (2004) *In Sickness and Wealth: The Corporate Assault on Global Health*, Boston, MA: South End Press.

Galtung, J. (2009) *The Fall of the US Empire – And Then What?*, Basel: Transcend University Press.

Glaser, W.A. (1993) 'The competition vogue and its outcomes', *The Lancet*, 341: 805–12.

Haines, A., Horton, R. and Bhutta, Z. (2007) 'Primary health care comes of age. Looking forward to the 30th anniversary of Alma-Ata: call for papers', *The Lancet*, 370: 911–13.

Harvey, D. (2005) *A Brief History of Neoliberalism*, Oxford: Oxford University Press.

Hermann, C. (2009) 'The marketization of health care in Europe', in L. Panitch and C. Leys (eds) *Morbid Symptoms: Health under Capitalism*, New York: Monthly Review Press.

Hunter, J.D. and Yates, J. (2002) 'In the vanguard of globalization: the world of American globalizers', in P.L. Berger and S.P. Huntington (eds), *Many Globalizations: Cultural Diversity in the Contemporary World*, Oxford and New York: Oxford University Press.

Jacobs, A. (1998) 'Seeing the difference: market health reform in Europe', *Journal of Health Politics, Policy and Law*, 23: 1–33.

Jacobson, B. (2010) 'Obama received $20 million from healthcare industry in 2008 campaign', *The Raw Story*. www.rawstory.com/rs/2010/01/12/obama-received-20-million-healthcare-industry-money-2008/

Jevons, W.J. (1911 [1970]) *The Theory of Political Economy*, Harmondsworth, UK: Penguin.

Johnson, C. (2004a) *Blowback: The Costs and Consequences of American Empire*, New York: Henry Holt.

——(2004b) *The Sorrows of Empire: Militarism, Secrecy, and the End of the Republic*, New York: Metropolitan Books.

——(2006) *Nemesis: The Last Days of the American Republic*, New York: Metropolitan Books.

Kickbusch, I. (2000) 'The development of international health policies – accountability intact?' *Social Science & Medicine*, 51: 979–89.

Kim, J.K., Joyce, V., Millen, J.V., Irwin, A. and Gershman, J. (eds) (2002) *Dying for Growth: Global Inequality and the Health of the Poor*, Monroe, ME: Common Courage Press.

Klein, N. (2007) *The Shock Doctrine: The Rise of Disaster Capitalism*, New York: Metropolitan.

Korten, D.C. (2001) *When Corporations Rule the World*, 2nd edn, San Francisco: Berrett-Koehler.

Laurell, A.C. (2003) 'What does Latin American social medicine do when it governs? The case of the Mexico City government', *American Journal of Public Health*, 93: 2028–31.

——(2007) 'Interview with Dr. Asa Cristina Laurell', *Social Medicine*, 2(1): 46–55.

——(2008) 'Health reform in Mexico City, 2000–2006', *Social Medicine*, 3(2): 145–57.

Lenin, V.I. (1917 [1963]) *Imperialism, the Highest Stage of Capitalism: A Popular Outline*, Moscow: Progress Publishers.

Levy, B.S. and Sidel, V.W. (eds) (2008) *War and Public Health*, Oxford and New York: Oxford University Press.

Light, D.W. (1997) 'Lessons for the United States: Britain's experience with managed competition', in J. D. Wilkinson, K.J. Devers and R.S. Givens (eds), *Competitive Managed Care: The Emerging Health Care System*, San Francisco, CA: Jossey-Bass.

Mackintosh, M. and Koivusalo, M. (eds) (2005) *Commercialization of Health Care: Global and Local Dynamics and Policy Responses*, New York: Palgrave Macmillan and United Nations Research Institute for Social Development.

Marshall, A. (1920 [1997]) *The Principles of Economics*, Amherst, NY: Prometheus Books.

Muntaner, C., Armada, F., Chung, H., Rosicar, M., Williams-Brennan, L. and Benach, J. (2008) 'Venezuela's Barrio Adentro: participatory democracy, south-south cooperation and health care for all', *Social Medicine*, 3: 232–46.

Navarro, V. (1974) 'The underdevelopment of health or the health of under-development: an analysis of the distribution of human health resources in Latin America', *Politics & Society*, 4: 267–93.

——(2007) (ed.) *Neoliberalism, Globalization, and Inequalities: Consequences for Health and Quality of Life*, Amityville, NY: Baywood.

Panitch, L. and Leys, C. (eds) (2009) *Morbid Symptoms: Health Under Capitalism*, New York: Monthly Review Press.

Price, D., Pollock, A.M. and Shaoul, J. (1999) 'How the World Trade Organization is shaping domestic policies in healthcare', *The Lancet*, 354: 1889–92.

Reid, T.R. (2009) *The Healing of America: A Global Quest for Better, Cheaper and Fairer Health Care*, New York: Penguin.

Ricardo, D. (1817 [1971]) *On the Principles of Political Economy and Taxation*, Harmondsworth, UK: Penguin.

Robinson, W.I. (2004) *A Theory of Global Capitalism: Production, Class, and State in a Transnational World*, Baltimore, MD: Johns Hopkins University Press.

——(2008) *Latin America and Global Capitalism: A Critical Globalization Perspective*, Baltimore, MD: Johns Hopkins University Press.

Romo, H.G. (1997) *La Contrarrevolución Neoliberal en México*, Mexico City: Ediciones Era.

Schuld, L. (2003a) 'El Salvador: who will have the hospitals?' *NACLA Report on the Americas*, 36(3): 42–45.

——(2003b) 'El Salvador: Anti-privatization victory', *NACLA Report on the Americas*, 37(1): 1.

Shaffer, E.R., Waitzkin, H., Jasso-Aguilar, R. and Brenner, J. (2005) 'Global trade and public health', *American Journal of Public Health*, 95: 23–34.

Silverman, M., Lydecker, M. and Lee, P.R. (1992) *Bad Medicine: The Prescription Drug Industry in the Third World*, Stanford, CA: Stanford University Press.

SIMETRISSS (2002) *Historical Agreement for the Betterment of the National Health System*, San Salvador, El Salvador: Sindicato Medico de Trabajadores del Instituto Salvadoreño del Seguro Social.

Smith, A. (1776 [1904]) *An Inquiry into the Nature and Causes of the Wealth of Nations*, London: Methuen.

STISSS (2002) *Chronology of the Movement*, San Salvador, El Salvador: Sindicato de Trabajadores del Instituto Salvadoreño del Seguro Social.

Stocker, K., Waitzkin, H. and Iriart, C. (1999) 'The exportation of managed care to Latin America', *New England Journal of Medicine*, 340: 1131–36.

Waitzkin, H. (2000) *The Second Sickness: Contradictions of Capitalist Health Care*, 2nd edn, Lanham, MD: Rowman & Littlefield.

——(2003) 'Report of the World Health Organization's Commission on Macroeconomics and Health – a summary and critique', *The Lancet*, 361: 523–26.

——(2011) *Medicine and Public Health at the End of Empire*, Boulder, CO: Paradigm Publishers.

Waitzkin, H., Iriart, C., Estrada, A. and Lamadrid, S. (2001a) 'Social medicine in Latin America: productivity and dangers facing the major national groups', *The Lancet*, 358: 315–23.

——(2001b) 'Social medicine then and now: lessons from Latin America', *American Journal of Public Health*, 91: 1592–1601.

Waitzkin, H., Jasso-Aguilar, R., Landwehr, A. and Mountain, C. (2005) 'Global trade, public health, and health services: stakeholders' constructions of the key issues', *Social Science & Medicine*, 61: 893–906.

Waitzkin, H., Jasso-Aguilar, R. and Iriart, C. (2007) 'Privatization of health services in less developed countries: an empirical response to the proposals of the World Bank and Wharton School', *International Journal of Health Services*, 37: 205–27.

Walras, L. (1984) *Elements of Pure Economics*, Philadelphia, PA: Orion Editions.

Woolhandler, S., Campbell, T. and Himmelstein, D.U. (2003) 'Costs of health care administration in the United States and Canada', *New England Journal of Medicine*, 349: 768–75.

Woolhandler, S., Day, B. and Himmelstein, D.U. (2008) 'State health reform flatlines', *International Journal of Health Services*, 38: 585–92.

Index

Page references in bold refer to a table and those in italics refer to a figure.

access to health care: community health
    service (Jinan City) 173–9, *177*, **178**;
    Mexico City 193–4; mixed private-
    public systems 200–1; Poland 123–5,
    125; primary care services 174; rights
    to (universal) 204–5; Russia 44–5, 48–9;
    as social right 194; USA 42, 200–1
activism 204–5
advertising campaigns (USA) 4, 8–9
ageing population 102, 103
ALBA (Bolivarian Alliance for the
    Peoples of Our America) 202
American Medical Association (AMA)
    4, 5–6, 13
America's Health Insurance Plans
    (AHIP) 11, 14–15
AMLO (Andrés Manuel López
    Obrador) 193, 194–5

backwardness versus modernity
    discourse 121–2, 125, 130–1, 133
Balcerowicz, Leszek 122, 123
Balicki, Marek 130
biopolitics 73–6
Blue Cross 5, 9
Blue Shield 5, 9
Bolivarian Alliance for the Peoples of
    Our America (ALBA) 202
Bourdieu, Pierre 204
Brazil 197
Bretton Woods accords 186–7

capitalism: and health care 186, 189–90;
    vulnerability of 203–4
Carnegie, Andrew 185
CEE countries (Central and Eastern
    Europe): mobility of health care

professionals 112–13; privatisation of
    health care 111–12; structural funds
    for health care 110–11
Chávez, Hugo 210
China: 'barefoot doctors' 77, 78;
    financing of health care system 171–2;
    health care campaigns 76–7; health
    care reforms 71, 72–3, 83, 164–6;
    health care within the service sector
    79–82; health insurance 80–1;
    informal payments to practitioners
    83, 84, 85, 87–8; as market economy
    75, 165; medical controversies 83–7;
    preventative health care 170; primary
    care services 165–7; public perception
    of health care professionals 71–2, 74,
    83; socialist health care system 76–8,
    86, 165; staff shortages 170–1;
    'stitched anus incident' 83–4;
    traditional Chinese medicine 76, 81,
    85, 86, 169; *yirenweiben* (human
    orientated) 82–3; *see also* community
    health service; Jinan City; *yihuan
    guanxi*
CHS (community health service) *see*
    community health service
citizenship, catastrophic 120–3, 125, 133
clinical commissioning groups (CCG)
    30–1
Clinton, William Jefferson "Bill" 7–9
collective health (Brazil) 197
commercialisation: health care
    provision (EU) 99–100, 102–4, 109–10,
    113–14; hospitals, Poland 128–30;
    see also privatisation of health care
community health service (CHS)
    (China): access to (Jinan City) 173–9,

177, **178**; challenges for 170–3, *173*; defined 166–7; development of 167–9, 172
Cuba 196, 202
cultural value of medical work 42–3, 47
Curtis, S. *et al.* 1995 46–7

data collection: financial 32; importance to health care planning 36–7; poor, by ISTCs 33; universal health systems 26–7
Davis, Dr (quoted) 62–4
democracy 125–6
dentistry (USA): community-based clinics 58–60; students 40, 41, 55, 57, 60–4; system 63–4
Devoted Dentists and Supporters (DDS) 61–2
disguising discourses 119, 126, 128, 133
doctors *see* physicians

El Salvador 191–3
empire: defined 182, 183; health care under 183–5; Latin American resistance to 190; weakness of 203; workers, health of 184, 186, 188–9
entitlement, sense of: patients 59–60; practitioners 41–2, 50, 54, 57, 60
Ernst & Young 131, 132
Europe, public-sector programs 198
European Commission, interest in health policies 97, 103–4, 105
European Court of Justice 97–8, 101–3
European Union: background and powers (box 5.1) 93–5; commercialisation of health care provision 99–100, 102–4, 109–10, 113–14; cross-border care 102, 103–4; Directive on Patients' Rights 103–4, 107; Directive on Services in the Internal Market 104; health services within Member States 102–8; health systems as basis for commercial growth 108–9; Lisbon Treaty (box 5.2) 95–7; open method of coordination (OMC) 100–1, 103; policy-making and health services 93, 95, 97–102; pre-authorisation for treatment 105, 106–7; relationship with CEE countries 110–13, 122–3

financial crisis: Europe 108, 111–12, 113; Hungary 143; Poland 118; Russia 46, 47

financing of health care systems: China 171–2; Hungary 140, 141–2 145-146, 147–9, 151–2; Mexico City 194–5; National Health Service (UK) 29–32; Poland 123, 128–9; Russia 45–7, 48–9
Foreign Direct Investment (FDI) 118, 122–3
Foucault, Michel 73–4
Fox, Vincente 193, 195

GATT (General Agreement on Tariffs and Trade) 187
Giza-Poleszczuk, Anna 120
Goldstein, H. and Spiegelhalter, D.J. 35

Health and Social Care Bill 25–6, 30–1
Health Care for American Now (HCAN) 11, 13
Healthcare Leadership Council (HLC) 8–9
health care planning 36
health care reforms: China 71, 72–3, 83, 164–6; Hungary 143–7; Russia 42, 43–4; USA 3–8, 10–16, 43; *see also* Patient Protection and Affordable Care Act
health care systems: as basis for commercial growth (EU) 108–9; China, socialist 76–8, 86, 165; comparisons 33–5; public option (USA) 10, 11–13, 14, 15; universal 26–7, 28, 36–7; worker productivity 183–5; *see also* market health care systems
health care workers: militarization of 184–5; social status of 50–4, 56–61, 71–2, 74, 87, 126–8; unionised 192–3
health geography 173–4
health insurance, private: Hungary 151; Poland 121, 130–2, 133; Russia 46, 48; United States of America 58
health insurance industry (USA): administration costs 199–200; America's Health Insurance Plans (AHIP) 11, 14–15; Healthcare Leadership Council (HLC) 8–9; opposition to medical reform 7–9, 11, 12–13, 14–16; and Patient Protection and Affordable Care Act 16–17, 200–2; population coverage 1, 5
health insurance plans (state): China 80–1; Hungary 140, 145, 147, *148*, 149, 151; Medicaid 6, 15, 55, 59, 60; Medicare 2, 11–12, 15, 199; Mexico 195; Poland 123; Russia (OMC) 45,

46, 48; single-payer universal 3–4,
198, 200
health maintenance organization
(HMO) 7, 11, 33–5
Hjertqvist, Johan 110
hospital privatisation: Hungary 151–7;
Poland 121, 128–30
Hu, President Jintao 82, 83
humanism: and biopolitics 75; *yihuan
guanxi* within 72–3, 82, 88; *yirenweiben*
(human orientated) 82–3
Hungary: civil society 158–9; current
health sector status 139–40; financing
of health care system 140, 141–2,
145–6, 147–9, 151–2; government and
electoral competition 159–60; health
care reforms 143–7; Health Insurance
Fund (HIF) 140, 145, 147, *148*, 149,
151; the 'Hospital Act' (2003) 153–7;
hospital privatisation 151–7; the
'Mikola Act' 151–3, 157–8; political
situation 141–4, 160; privatisation of
health care 140, 141, 143–4, 149–51,
153–8

Ignagni, Karen 11, 13
independent sector treatment centres
(ISTC) 32–3
infectious diseases 77, 186, 188–9
informal payments from patients
(China) 83, 84, 85, 87–8
informal payments from patients
(Russia) 49, 51, 52
information systems 25
insurance companies *see* health
insurance industry (USA)
international financial institutions 186–7
international health organizations 188–90
International Monetary Fund (IMF)
122, 187, 197, 201
International Sanitary Bureau 188–9
international trade agreements 187–8, 202
ISSS (Salvadoran Institute of Social
Security) 191–3
Iurin, Andrei 49–50

Jinan City: access to community health
service (study) 173–5; access to
community health service (study)
results 176–9, *177*, **178**; background
to 175; methodological approach to
study 175–6
Johnson, Lyndon 6
journalism, standards 21–2

Kaiser Permanente 33–5
Kennedy, Ted (Edward Moore) 7

labour force, health of 184, 186, 188–9
Latin America 190, 198, 201, 202–3
Laurell, Christina 193–4
Lenin, Vladimir Ilyich 203
Lisbon Treaty 95–7 (box 5.2), 103
López Obrador, Andrés Manuel
(AMLO) 193, 194–5
Luntz, Frank 10

managed care 20, 197–8
managed care organization (MCO)
197, 198
market health care systems:
assumptions of efficiency of (EU)
101; inequalities of (China) 85, 165–6;
inequalities of (USA) 1–2, 43; moral
economies 43, 58; political support
for 199; resource allocation 30–1;
risk-allocation 25, 28–9; risk-selection
25–8, 33–6
MCG (Mexico City Government) 193–5
Medicaid 6, 15, 55, 59, 60, 64
medical loss ratio (MLR) 1
Medical Union of Workers of the
Salvadoran Institute of Social
Security (SIMETRISSS) 192–3
Medicare 2, 5–6, 10–12, 15, 199
memories: communist health care
system (China) 78; socialist health
care system (Poland) 126–8
Mercosur 202
Mexico City, health policies in 193–5
Mexico City Government (MCG) 193–5
MLR (medical loss ratio) 1
moral economies: defined 41; as
framework for analysis 66; market
health care systems 43, 58;
professional entitlement 60–4;
Russian health workers 47–8, 50,
51–2; workforce trends (USA) 55–60
mortality rates: as measure of hospital
quality 35; Poland 118; Russia
(1990s) 44

National Health Service (NHS):
administrative structures 25–6;
area-based funding 29–30; capital
funding 31–2; geographic base 26, 28,
36; Health and Social Care Bill 25–6;
Private Finance Initiative (PFI) 31–2, 128
National Health Service Corps (NHSC) 55

neofunctionalism 98
neoliberalism 75, 182–3, 193, 195
Nixon, Richard 7, 55

Obama, Barack, health care reform 1–2,
    10–16, 56, 198–201
OMC (open method of coordination)
    (EU) 100–1
OMC (quasi-governmental insurance
    fund) (Russia) 45, 46, 48

Pachocki, Robert 124
Palin, Sarah 10
Pan American Health Organization
    (PAHO) 189
Patient Protection and Affordable Care
    Act: development of 10–16, 198–9;
    insurance industry's response to
    16–17, 200–2; and primary care 56;
    responses to 18–21
pharmaceutical industry 99–100, 118,
    123–4, 129, 184
philanthropic foundations 185–6
planning systems, data collection 27
Poland: access to health care 123–5,
    125; dependent development
    (economic) 122–3, 133; financing of
    health care system 123, 128–9;
    hospital privatisation 121, 128–30;
    liberalism 119, 121, 132; *mohery* 119;
    pharmaceutical industry 118, 123–4,
    129; political economy of shame xii,
    130–1; post-socialist state 121–2;
    private health insurance 121, 130–2,
    133; public mourning 119–20;
    socialist health care system 126–8;
    social modernity and citizens 125–6,
    131–2, 133; societal exclusion, sense
    of 120–1; true citizens 126, 131;
    underserved communities 118;
    Universal Health Insurance 123
politics, and health policy: China 72, 79,
    83; Hungary 143–7, 149; Poland
    121–3, 130–2; *see also* empire;
    European Union; health care
    reforms; privatisation of health care
PricewaterhouseCoopers (PwC)
    14–15
primary care services: access to 174;
    Hungary 146; low numbers workers
    55–6; low prestige of 56–60; moral
    economies 60–1; underdevelopment
    of (China) 165–7; United States of
    America 55–8, 59, 65; Venezuela

1960s; WHO mandate 189; *see also*
    community health service
Private Finance Initiatives (PFI) 31–2,
    128
privatisation of health care: CEE
    countries 111–12; El Salvador,
    attempted 191–3; Hungary 140, 141,
    143–4, 149–51, 153–8; Poland 121,
    128–30; *see also* commercialisation
public health care: assumption of poor
    physician skills 40–1, 43, 47; Brazil
    197; effect of trade agreements 202;
    El Salvador 191–3; Mexico City
    193–5; popularity of in Europe 198;
    Uruguay 196–7; Venezuela 196
public option, health care reform
    (USA) 10, 11–13, 14, 15
public relations (USA) 2–3, 4–5, 21–2
public relations, stealth PR xi–xii, 3
Putin, Vladimir 43, 44

reform and remuneration 64–5
risk analyses: allocation 28–9; capital
    planning 31–2; identification 27–8,
    33; and patient selection 32–3;
    pooling 28; resource allocation 29–32;
    selection 33–7
Robinson, William 204–5
Rockefeller Foundation 185–6
Russia: access to health care 44–5, 48–9;
    health care financing models 45–7,
    48–9; health care reforms 42, 43–4;
    informal payments to practitioners
    49, 51, 52; National Project for health
    care 44; physician's remuneration
    40–1, 42–3, 45, 49–54, 65

Salvadoran Institute of Social Security
    (ISSS) 191–3
SARS (severe acute respiratory
    syndrome) xi, xii, 72, 166, 168
Sawicka, Beata (quoted) 129
scandals, medical: China 83–6; Poland
    129–30
schistosomiasis 77
Schwarzenegge, Arnold 20
Shanghai 79–80, 87
Silva, Luiz Inácio Lula da (Lula) 197
SIMETRISSS (Medical Union of
    Workers of the Salvadoran Institute
    of Social Security) 192–3
single-payer universal health care 3–4,
    198, 200
Skocpol, Theda 9

socialized medicine 4–5, 6
social status, health care workers 50–4,
   56–61, 71–2, 74, 87, 126–8
sociomedical activisim 204
surgery, elective, contracted out (UK) 33
symbolic capital 57
symbolic violence 133
Sztompka, Piotr 122, 125–6

tobacco companies 2–3
Truman, Harry S. 3–4, 6
Twigg, Judyth 46, 47

underdevelopment of health 183–4
underserved communities: dentistry
   (USA) 58–60; Poland 118; primary
   care for (USA) 55–6, 59, 65
United Nations 189
United States of America: access to
   health care 42, 200–1; death panels
   10, 14; decline traditional journalism
   21–2; government takeover 10–11, 12;
   Health Care for American Now
   (HCAN) 11; health care reforms 3–8,
   10–16, 43; health maintenance
   organization (HMO) 7; inadequacies
   of health system 1–2, 43; managed
   care 20, 197–8; political campaign
   funding 17–18; primary care 55–8, 59,
   65; public health mentality 59; public
   relations campaigns 2–3; relationship
   with Latin America 190;
   remuneration for practitioners 40, 41,
   57, 58–9; social status health care

workers 56–61; Tea Party 11; *see also*
   health insurance industry (USA);
   Patient Protection and Affordable
   Care Act
universal health systems: administrative
   functions 26–7; geographic function
   26, 28, 36–7; risk-pooling 28
Uruguay 196–7

Venezuela 196, 203
volunteers: dental students 58–9, 61–2;
   standards of care 40, 41, 58–9

Washington Consensus 183, 187
Wikileaks 130
Wolff, Larry 122
workers, health of 184, 186, 188–9
World Bank 187, 189, 193, 201
World Health Organization (WHO) 77,
   81, 166, 167, 170, 189–90
World Trade Organization (WTO)
   187–8, 202

yihuan guanxi (relations between medical
   professionals and patients):
   biopolitical analysis 74, 75–6; and
   humanism 72–3, 82, 88; inequality of
   doctor-patient relationship 85–7;
   interview with Dr Xuemin 71–2; and
   medical scandals 84–5; and socialist
   health care system 78

Zalicki, Łukasz 131
Zhang, Wenkang 72